Handbook of Coronary Care

Sixth Edition

Joseph S. Alpert, M.D.
Robert S. and Irene P. Flinn Chair of Medicine
College of Medicine
Department of Medicine
The University of Arizona Health Sciences Center
Tucson, Arizona

Gary S. Francis, M.D.
Director, Coronary Intensive Care Unit
Department of Cardiology
The Cleveland Clinic Foundation
Cleveland, Ohio

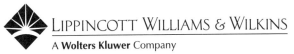

LIPPINCOTT WILLIAMS & WILKINS
A **Wolters Kluwer** Company

Philadelphia · Baltimore · New York · London
Buenos Aires · Hong Kong · Sydney · Tokyo

Acquisitions Editor: Ruth W. Weinberg
Developmental Editor: Anjou K. Dargar
Production Editor: Emily Lerman
Manufacturing Manager: Colin J. Warnock
Cover Designer: Jeane Norton
Compositor: Circle Graphics
Printer: Vicks Lithographers

© 2000 by LIPPINCOTT WILLIAMS & WILKINS
530 Walnut Street
Philadelphia, PA 19106 USA
LWW.com

Library of Congress Cataloging-in-Publication Data

Alpert, Joseph S.
    Handbook of coronary care / Joseph S. Alpert, Gary S. Francis.—6th ed.
        p. ; cm.
    Includes bibliographical references and index.
    ISBN 0-7817-1958-5 (alk. paper)
        1. Coronary heart disease—Handbooks, manuals, etc. I. Francis, Gary S.,
    1943- II. Title.
        [DNLM: 1. Coronary Disease—Handbook. WG 39 A333m 2000]
    RC685.C6 A515 2000
    616.1′23—dc21

                                                                                    00-022471

This book is dedicated to our parents and teachers, without whom it would never have been started; and to our wives, without whom it would never have been finished.

Contents

Preface

Remarkable advances have occurred in the field of coronary care since we wrote the first edition of this book in 1976. At that time, infarct size reduction was still an experimental idea and thrombolysis had hardly been conceived. In that era, patients were kept in a quiet, darkened environment and arrhythmia treatment and prevention represented the cornerstone of coronary care. Today, thrombolysis and infarct size and prevention are the standard of care for patients with acute coronary syndromes, i.e., myocardial infarction and unstable angina. The five previous editions of *Handbook of Coronary Care* have witnessed the evolution of coronary care from a mostly passive, supportive endeavor to the modern, aggressive approach employed today. This sixth edition contains new material that will assist physicians and nurses in caring for patients with acute coronary syndromes. Two new chapters discuss hyperlipidemia and sexuality in the coronary patient. The other 31 chapters and appendices have been extensively updated and revised. However, we continue to use the original style that has been so successful in the past: introductory remarks followed by a concise series of recommendations listed in guideline format, and finally, a current, concise bibliography.

As in the previous five editions, we present our own particular approach to each problem founded on evidence-based principles. We recognize that there are alternative strategies in the management of patients with acute coronary syndromes and that not every authority will agree with all of our recommendations. Nevertheless, we feel that our suggestions represent solid ground from which to begin a discussion of the various diagnostic and therapeutic approaches to these patients.

Joseph S. Alpert, M.D.
Gary S. Francis, M.D.

Acknowledgments

The authors acknowledge the inspiration and assistance of the following individuals: James E. Dalen, M.D., Gordon Ewy, M.D., and Steven Goldman, M.D., of the University of Arizona; Eric Topol, M.D., of the Cleveland Clinic; Joel M. Gore, M.D. and Richard Becker, M.D., of the University of Massachusetts; Jay N. Cohn, M.D., of the University of Minnesota; Eugene Braunwald, M.D., Eliot Antman, M.D., and Bernard Lown, M.D., of Brigham and Women's Hospital; Robert A. O'Rourke, M.D., of the University of Texas at San Antonio. We are most appreciative of the editorial support of Anjou K. Dargar and Ruth W. Weinberg of Lippincott Williams & Wilkins.

Handbook of Coronary Care

Sixth Edition

1

Introduction to the CCU

Coronary care units (CCUs) were first organized to monitor patients with acute myocardial infarction (AMI) and to treat the lethal ventricular arrhythmias to which these patients are prone. This goal of the CCU has been generally achieved, with a consequent reduction in the acute mortality of patients with MI. The residual mortality in AMI is related to the extent of damage that the infarcted heart sustains. Efforts in the field of coronary care, in addition to understanding and treating arrhythmias, are now focused on reducing the amount of myocardial necrosis in an attempt to limit left ventricular dysfunction and resultant mortality from cardiogenic shock.

Myocardial infarction results when myocardial cells receive insufficient blood-borne nutrients and oxygen, usually as a result of coronary thrombosis. Other myocardial cells, both adjacent to and sometimes remote from the center of cell necrosis, are rendered severely ischemic by the same process that caused the MI. Damage to the latter cells may not be irreversible, and the focus of modern coronary care is therapy that will permit salvage of this reversibly injured myocardium.

Most interventions that reduce the demand of myocardial cells for nutrients (especially oxygen) will be of benefit to ischemic myocardium. However, a reduction in myocardial oxygen demand can be detrimental if, for example, it is associated with an arterial pressure inadequate to perfuse segments of the coronary circulation distal to occlusive lesions. Thus, if arterial diastolic pressure is reduced to 60 mm Hg or less, there may be greater myocardial ischemia despite a reduction in myocardial oxygen demand.

Myocardial oxygen consumption has three major determinants: heart rate, myocardial contractility (the strength and vigor of myocardial contraction), and ventricular wall stress. Ventricular wall stress is related to ventricular cavity size and intraventricular pressure. Thus, both ventricular dilatation and left ventricular hypertension increase left ventricular wall stress, and hence myocardial oxygen consumption. Another way of conceptualizing myocardial oxygen demand also involves three variables: heart rate, preload or end-diastolic fiber length (directly proportional to end-diastolic left ventricular volume), and afterload or left ventricular systolic wall tension (related to left ventricular systolic pressure).

Extensive ventricular myocardial necrosis and/or ischemia predispose the patient to heart failure, arrhythmias, and other complications of MI. Physicians writing orders for patients with acute MI should constantly ask themselves this question: Is this particular intervention going to aid in reducing the patient's myocardial oxygen demand and/or increase myocardial blood flow?

Much attention has focused on ways to dissolve the coronary arterial thrombus that has interrupted myocardial blood flow. Pharmacologic (thrombolytic) and mechanical (angioplasty) techniques are both successful in removing the offending thrombus. Prevention of coronary arterial thrombosis would, of course, be preferable to dissolution of an already established thrombosis. However, the exact sequence of events leading to coronary thrombosis is still being intensely studied.

Most patients with coronary arterial thrombosis and AMI have underlying coronary arterial atherosclerosis. Most often, individuals develop thrombosis in relation to an atherosclerotic plaque that is not obstructing coronary blood flow. In these latter patients, plaque rupture and sometimes coronary artery spasm cause coronary thrombosis despite the absence of a high-grade obstructing lesion in the coronary arterial tree. Spasm may disrupt a minor atherosclerotic plaque, leading to a fissure in the plaque, with resultant exposure of underlying tissue elements to the circulating blood. Alternatively, spasm might reduce the rate of blood flow in an artery, leading to zones of stagnant flow. Both of these mechanisms, working separately or together, would increase the likelihood that a coronary arterial thrombus would form. Other potential mechanisms leading to coronary thrombosis include plaque rupture secondary to stress fatigue or biochemical dissolution of structural proteins and/or collagen by inflammatory cells (e.g., macrophages) working within the atherosclerotic plaque itself.

Once thrombosis has occurred, survival of the myocardial zone supplied by the thrombosed artery depends on (a) collateral blood flow that bypasses the obstructed arterial segment and (b) myocardial oxygen demand. When blood supply, oxygen demand, or both exceed certain limits, myocardial cell necrosis is initiated. Myocardial necrosis starts approximately 20 minutes after coronary arterial thrombosis and proceeds in a wave front from the subendocardium to the epicardium. Myocardial cell death becomes more or less transmural in extent approximately 3–4 hours following coronary thrombosis if collateral blood flow is absent. Thus, measures to reopen the obstructed artery should begin as quickly as possible. In the clinical setting, myocardial necrosis is said to begin when the patient first notes ischemic pain that is unrelieved by nitroglycerin or other maneuvers (such as lying down). Chapters 12 and 13 outline measures that are currently used to decrease infarct size by increasing myocardial blood flow and decreasing myocardial oxygen demand. Hopefully, future investigation will give us sufficient insight into the exact nature of the pathophysiologic sequence that leads to coronary arterial thrombosis so that it can be prevented. Until then, we must strive to keep each MI as small as possible.

BIBLIOGRAPHY

Buja, L.M., and Entman, M.L. Modes of myocardial cell injury and cell death in ischemic heart disease. *Circulation* 98:1355–1357, 1998.

Dunn, R.F., Botvinick, E.H., Benge, W., Chatterjee, K., and Parmley, W.W. The significance of nitroglycerin-induced changes in ventricular function after acute myocardial infarction. *Am. J. Cardiol.* 49:1719–1727, 1982.

Jennings, R.B., and Reimer, K.A. Salvage of ischemic myocardium. *Mod. Concepts Cardiovasc. Dis.* 43:125–130, 1974.

Kullo, I.J., Edwards, W.D., and Schwartz, R.S. Vulnerable plaque: Pathobiology and clinical implications. *Ann. Intern. Med.* 129:1050–1060, 1998.

Lau, J., Antman, E.M., Jimenez-Silva, J., et al. Cumulative meta-analysis of therapeutic trials for myocardial infarction. *N. Engl. J. Med.* 327:248–254, 1992.

Muller, J.E., Kaufmann, P.G., Luepker, R.V., Weisfeldt, M.L., Deedwania, P.C., and Willerson, J.T. Mechanisms precipitating acute cardiac events: Review and recommendations of an NHLBI workshop. *Circulation* 96:3233–3239, 1997.

Simoons, M.L., et al. Early thrombolysis in acute myocardial infarction: Limitation of infarct size and improved survival. *J. Am. Coll. Cardiol.* 7:717–728, 1986.

Sonnenblick, E.H., and Skelton, C.L. Oxygen consumption of the heart: Physiological principles and clinical implications. *Mod. Concepts Cardiovasc. Dis.* 40:9–16, 1971.

Yusuf, S., Sleight, P., Held, P., McMahon, S. Routine medical management of acute myocardial infarction—Lessons from overviews of recent randomized controlled trials. *Circulation* 82(suppl. II):II-117–II-134, 1990.

2

The CCU Environment

Patients admitted to a coronary care unit (CCU) with an acute myocardial infarction (AMI) are almost invariably distraught. Frequently, the physiologic concomitants of this emotional state are elevated blood pressure and elevated pulse. Increases in heart rate and left ventricular pressure result in increased myocardial oxygen demand (see Chapter 1). Increases in myocardial oxygen demand can increase myocardial ischemia and necrosis (see Fig. 12.1).

Considerable evidence points to a central nervous system origin for a substantial portion of the ventricular arrhythmias associated with AMI. This "hypothalamic" origin of ventricular arrhythmias is felt to be mediated through excessive or unopposed sympathetic nerve stimulation. In particular, ventricular arrhythmias occurring early in the course of acute MI are mediated by the central nervous system. It is of interest that some of these ventricular arrhythmias are resistant to lidocaine suppression while often responding to beta blockade.

Experimental as well as clinical observations document the importance of psychological factors in the generation of cardiac arrhythmias. These arrhythmias may result from the combination of an unstable electrical milieu in the myocardium, together with centrally mediated excessive or unopposed sympathetic nerve stimulation secondary to emotional upset.

For these reasons, it is mandatory that the CCU environment combat the psychological trauma and the emotionally distraught state occurring in most patients with AMI. Certain rules are axiomatic:

1. Quiet, confident, and generally serious (but not funereal) demeanor is necessary at all times in the CCU. This mental state is required of all who work in the CCU:

    *   physicians
    *   nurses
    *   aides and
    *   secretaries

2. It is important to communicate to the patient (by word, deed, and demeanor) that everything is under control. A careful explanation of the purpose of the various moni-

toring devices is invaluable in this regard. It is important to stress to patients that the monitoring equipment protects them during the acute phase of the MI.

3. Conferences with colleagues, consultants, medical students, and others should be held out of the patient's hearing range. Gestures or expressions that might be misinterpreted by the patient should be avoided. Moreover, daily, supportive contact with the patient is essential.

4. Information given to a patient's family should be straightforward but nonetheless as encouraging as possible without glossing over potential risks. Most hospitals require that patients admitted to the CCU be classified as seriously ill or critical. The reasons for this and its implications should be explained to family members. Physicians and nurses should try to be as positive and confident with the patient as the situation allows, without becoming superficial or flippant.

5. Procedures that are deemed necessary (e.g., cardioversion, catheter insertion) should be explained carefully to the patient. Risk should be mentioned but not overemphasized.

6. A mild sedative (e.g., alprazolam) and a sleeping medication (e.g., flurazepam) are usually prescribed for patients in the CCU unless contraindicated (e.g., in chronic obstructive pulmonary disease with CO_2 retention).

7. When patients are transferred from the CCU to another part of the hospital, the positive aspect of this transfer (i.e., the fact that recovery is sufficiently advanced to allow the patient to leave the CCU) should be emphasized. Patients should be warned early in the course of their CCU admission that they may be moved at any time and that this move does not represent a compromise in their care.

8. Daily contact with the outside world is important for the patient in order to prevent the development of the "ICU syndrome," a confused and agitated state of consciousness said to be related to sensory deprivation, which can occur in intensive care units. Thus, daily newspapers and visitors are encouraged; each room contains a calendar and a clock as well a radio and television set, but stimulating forms of entertainment such as televised sporting events should be curtailed. Patients and visitors are strongly advised to refrain from stressful business or personal discussions and activities. Limited telephone use is allowed.

9.   Early contact with cardiac rehabilitation staff is recommended.

BIBLIOGRAPHY

Cassem, N.H., and Hackett, T.P. Psychiatric consultation in a coronary care unit. *Ann. Intern. Med.* 75:9–14, 1971.

Ford, D.E., Mead, L.A., Chang, P.P., Cooper-Patrick, L., Wang, N.Y., and Klag, M.J. Depression is a risk factor for coronary artery disease in men. *Arch. Intern. Med.* 158: 1422–1426, 1998.

Hackett, T.P., and Cassem, N.H. *Coronary Care: Patient Psychology.* New York and Dallas: American Heart Association, 1975.

Hackett, T.P., Cassem, N.H., and Wishne, H.A. The coronary care unit: An appraisal of its psychologic hazards. *N. Engl. J. Med.* 279:1365–1370, 1968.

Lear, M.W. *Heartsounds.* New York: Simon & Schuster, 1980.

Lown, B., and Verrier, R.L. Neural activity and ventricular fibrillation. *N. Engl. J. Med.* 294:1165–1170, 1976.

Lynch, J.J., Paskewitz, D.A., Gimbel, K.S., and Thomas, S.A. Psychological aspects of cardiac arrhythmia. *Am. Heart J.* 93:645–657, 1977.

Skinner, J.E. Regulation of cardiac vulnerability by the cerebral defense system *J. Am. Coll. Cardiol.* 5:88B–94B, 1985.

3

The CCU Nurse

Nowhere else in the hospital does the nurse have as much responsibility or act as independently as in the coronary care unit (CCU). Coronary care nurses should all be specially trained in the recognition and treatment of arrhythmias. They should also be adroit at managing hemodynamic monitoring systems. They should be encouraged to keep current by reading, attending meetings, and so on. They are constantly in the presence of the patients in the CCU, and it is the coronary care nurse who is largely responsible for creating the necessary special environment (see Chapter 2).

Some physicians, particularly early in their training, feel threatened by coronary care nurses because of the nurses' superior expertise in dealing with cardiac arrhythmias. Such feelings on the part of physicians are usually unjustified, and learning to cope with them is part of the physician's job. Coronary care nurses, while justifiably proud of their special abilities, are anxious to help physicians who are new to the CCU. This help is usually offered in an unobtrusive and hence nonthreatening manner, and physicians inexperienced in coronary care should avail themselves of the expertise of the coronary care nurse without feeling in any way diminished.

Hospitals differ in the extent to which they allow coronary care nurses freedom of action. In some institutions, nurses are allowed to initiate treatment with a variety of intravenous medicines (e.g., lidocaine, atropine, morphine, pressors), according to fixed protocols. All hospitals allow CCU nurses to perform defibrillation. House officers as well as staff physicians should know what the CCU nurses in their particular institution can and cannot do. Such an awareness prevents embarrassing, time-consuming, and divisive arguments.

It should be axiomatic in all CCUs that physicians and nurses work together harmoniously to create the required environment (see Chapter 2).

4

Transfer of Patients to the CCU

Potentially fatal ventricular bradyarrhythmias and tachy-arrhythmias commonly occur in the early phase (first few hours) of acute myocardial infarction (AMI). Patients with MI are usually first seen in a triage or emergency care area. Thus, it is not uncommon for patients with acute MI to have ventricular arrhythmias during their stay in the triage or emergency area. Occasionally, patients have dangerous arrhythmias during transport from the triage or emergency area to the coronary care unit (CCU). It is therefore important that patients be transferred to the CCU rapidly. Certain important precautions should be taken during this transfer:

PROTOCOL

1. A physician and/or nurse (or competent technician, licensed practical nurse, or aide trained in cardiopulmonary resuscitation) should accompany the patient during transfer.
2. The patient should be connected to a portable monitor with a clear electrocardiographic (ECG) tracing visible on the screen.
3. The patient should have a stable intravenous line (preferably a plastic cannula and not just a scalp-vein needle) in place and running at a very slow rate; 5% D/W should be used as the infusate.
4. The following should accompany the patient during transfer:
    a. A portable, battery-operated defibrillator.
    b. Two syringes with needles in place, one containing 100 mg of lidocaine and the other containing 1 mg of atropine.
5. The patient should receive nasal oxygen from a portable oxygen tank during transfer.
6. Transfer should be as rapid as is safely possible.
7. The emergency room staff should telephone the CCU staff and advise them of the imminent arrival of the patient. This call should be made before the patient leaves the emergency room to ensure that a bed is available.

INTERHOSPITAL TRANSFERS OF PATIENTS WITH ACUTE MYOCARDIAL INFARCTION

Early intervention for reduction of infarct size with mechanical or pharmacologic thrombolytic therapy, intravenous nitroglycerin, and beta blockade requires that the patient be admitted to a CCU that is conversant with such interventions. These units are usually directed by one or more cardiologists who are constantly available and are often employed full or part time by the hospital. Catheterization and angioplasty services are also usually required to support such early intervention protocols (see Chapters 13, 28, and 30).

Although aggressive management strategies—such as thrombolytic therapy, intravenous beta blockers, and nitroglycerin—are employed in community hospitals without full-time cardiology departments, some patients who receive these therapies will require transfer to a tertiary care center at some point during their hospital course for further invasive evaluation and possibly angioplasty or coronary bypass surgery. Some physicians prefer to transfer all younger individuals who present in the early stages of an AMI to a tertiary care center. Intravenous thrombolytic therapy is usually initiated immediately prior to the transfer. Some physicians prefer to administer thrombolytic agents in the community hospital setting with subsequent transfer to the tertiary care center 2 to 3 days later for catheterization and possible angioplasty.

Regardless of the exact timing of the transfers, all of these patients will have had a recent MI. Transfers should be made by specially equipped ambulance or helicopter with special precautions taken (e.g., monitoring, potential for defibrillation, and resuscitation). Equipment for and personnel conversant with American Heart Association Advanced Cardiac Life Support (ACLS) must be present during transfers. Often an ACLS-certified nurse and a physician accompany patients. Other medical systems employ one or two ACLS nurses or emergency medical technicians without a physician for interhospital transfers of patients with AMI. The following equipment and personnel are recommended:

PROTOCOL

1. At least one, preferably two, ACLS-certified medical personnel, one of whom is often a physician.
2. Equipment for ACLS support of patients includes:
   a. Endotracheal intubation equipment, i.e., laryngoscope; various-sized endotracheal tubes; tank of sup-

plemental oxygen; a manual bag-valve-mask resuscitator with different-sized masks, oral airways, and bite sticks; and tubing to connect the oxygen supply to the resuscitator or face masks.

b. Portable suction.

c. Full complement of intravenous fluids and drugs such as atropine, lidocaine, isoproterenol, epinephrine, calcium chloride, sodium bicarbonate, dopamine, dobutamine, amrinone, furosemide, nitroglycerin, nitroprusside, propranolol or metoprolol, procainamide, bretylium, diazepam, morphine, and heparin.

d. Equipment for ECG and hemodynamic monitoring.

e. DC current cardioverter/defibrillator.

f. Equipment for introduction of intravenous cannulae or needles under sterile conditions, i.e., sterile gauze, Betadine swabs, intravenous needles and cannulae, and suturing equipment.

g. Temporary pacemaker, intravenous or external.

h. Pericardiocentesis kit.

3. Prior to patient transport, the following general measures should be taken:

a. Secure airway patency.

b. Secure intravenous infusions and be sure adequate fluid is available in plastic bags for the duration of the transport. Two intravenous lines should be available for all patients.

c. Ensure that supplemental inspiratory oxygen is reaching the patient.

4. It is important to bear in mind that ACLS-level resuscitation may be required during transport.

BIBLIOGRAPHY

Braman, S.S., Dunn, S.M., Amico, C.A., and Millman, R.P. Complications of intrahospital transport in critically ill patients. *Ann. Intern. Med.* 107:469–473, 1987.

Gore, J.M., Corrao, J.M., Goldberg, R.J., et al. Feasibility and safety of emergency interhospital transport of patients during early hours of acute myocardial infarction. *Arch. Intern. Med.* 149:353–355, 1989.

Task Force of the European Society of Cardiology and The European Resuscitation Council: The pre-hospital management of acute heart attacks. *Eur. Heart J.* 19:1140–1164, 1998.

Textbook of Advanced Cardiac Life Support (2nd ed.). New York and Dallas: American Heart Association, 1990.

5

Prognosis in Acute Myocardial Infarction

The skill required to determine the prognosis of an individual patient is one of the more important spheres of knowledge that a physician can master. It requires considerable insight regarding the natural history of the disease, both treated and untreated. Patients and their families can never seem to get enough information about prognosis.

Historically, prior to the thrombolytic era, the Killip classification was used to help determine the prognosis of patients with acute myocardial infarction (AMI). It was developed by Dr. Thomas Killip and colleagues at the then Myocardial Infarction Research Unit of the New York Hospital/Cornell University Medical Center in the 1960s, and is still used today in discussing short-term prognosis:

The Killip classification is as follows:

Class I: No heart failure; mortality ~ 2% to 6%
Class II: Mild to moderate heart failure (S_3, rales no more than halfway up the back); mortality ~ 10% to 20%
Class III: Severe heart failure (pulmonary edema); mortality ~ 30% to 40%
Class IV: Cardiogenic shock; mortality ≥ 50%

The thrombolytic era was ushered in during the 1980s and reduced the overall acute hospital mortality for AMI from ~ 15% to ~ 7.5%, a remarkable advance. The outlook for patients with cardiogenic shock has remained grim but has been improved by primary angioplasty/stenting (see Chapter 21). Patients presenting with heart failure continue to have a high mortality. Using the large population of the international Global Utilization of Streptokinase and Tissue plasminogen activator for Occluded coronary arteries (GUSTO-I) trial (41,021 patients admitted to 1,081 hospitals in 15 countries), a comprehensive analysis of associations between baseline clinical variables and 30-day mortality after thrombolytic therapy has been performed using a multivariate statistical model. Age continues to be the most important clinical factor, with mortality rates of 1.1% in the youngest decile (< 45 years) and 20.5% in patients > 75 years ($p < 0.0001$). Other important variables include low systolic blood pressure ($p < 0.0001$), higher Killip class ($p < 0.0001$),

Table 5-1.   Comparison of anterior and inferior myocardial infarction

Pathology	Anterior MI	Inferior MI
Extent of necrosis	Greater than inferior MI	Less than anterior MI
Extent of coronary artherosclerosis	Less than inferior MI	Greater than anterior MI
Complications		
• Ventricular septal rupture	Apical, more easily repaired	Basal, more difficult to repair
• Aneurysm	Common	Uncommon
• Free wall rupture	Uncommon	Very uncommon
• Papillary muscle rupture	Anterolateral papillary muscle, rare	Posteromedial papillary muscle, less rare; right ventricular papillary muscle, very rare
• Mural thrombus	More common than with inferior MI	Less common than with anterior MI
Prognosis		
• Overall	Worse than that of inferior MI	Better than that of anterior MI
• In hospital	Worse than that of inferior MI	Better than that of anterior MI
Diagnosis		
• Presentation	Gastrointestinal symptoms unusual	Gastrointestinal symptoms (nausea, vomiting, hiccough) common
• Physical examination	Bradycardia; hypotension uncommon	Bradycardia; hypotension common
	Jugular venous distention less common than with inferior MI	Jugular venous distention more common than with anterior MI
	50% have S_3	20% have S_3

• Electrocardiogram	Sinus tachycardia more commonly observed than with inferior MI	Sinus bradycardia more commonly observed than with anterior MI
	Supraventricular arrhythmia secondary to left ventricular failure; mortality increased	Supraventricular arrhythmia secondary to ischemia of sinus node or increased vagal tone; mortality not increased
	First-degree A-V block often the result of block below His bundle	First-degree A-V block often the result of block above His bundle
	Mobitz type II, second-degree A-V block more common than with inferior MI; complete heart block often follows Mobitz type II A-V block	Mobitz type I, second-degree A-V block more common than with anterior MI; complete heart block rarely follows Mobitz type I A-V block
	Complete heart block is sudden in onset, followed by idioventriclar escape rhythm, and carries a high mortality rate (70–80%)	Complete heart block is gradual in onset, followed by nodal escape rhythm, and carries a relatively low mortality rate (20–25%)
	RBBB more common than in inferior MI	
• Radionuclide ventriculogram or echocardiography	Abnormal left ventricular wall motion is anterior in location and more severe than in inferior MI; no abnormal right ventricular wall motion	Abnormal left ventricular wall motion is inferior in location and less severe than in anterior MI; right ventricular abnormal wall motion present in approximately one-third of patients

MI, myocardial infarction; A-V, atrioventricular; RBBB, right bundle branch block.
(From Alpert JS. A comparison of anterior and inferior myocardial infarction. In: Rippe JM, Irwin RS, Alpert JS, Dalen JE, eds. *Intensive Care Medicine* 2nd ed. Boston: Little, Brown, 1991. With permission.)

elevated heart rate or bradycardia, and anterior MI. These five variables contained 90% of the 30-day prognostic information. **Blood pressure was highly important and, somewhat surprisingly, prognosis began to worsen as systolic blood pressure fell below 120 mm Hg.** Other though less important prognostic variables include previous MI, previous bypass surgery, diabetes mellitus, time to treatment, height, weight, type of thrombolytic, and a history of hypertension or prior cerebrovascular accident.

Just as it is important to identify high-risk patients following AMI, it is equally if not more important to identify low-risk patients. Early cardiac catheterization and careful observation can identify patients who are likely to be free from late major complications:

1. Absence of early sustained ventricular tachycardia
2. Absence of early ventricular fibrillation
3. Absence of early sustained hypotension
4. Absence of cardiogenic shock
5. Fewer coronary arteries with 75% stenosis or less
6. Preserved left ventricular ejection fraction

The first 24–48 hours is the period of highest risk. Patients with no complications within the first 24 hours after infarction can sometimes be moved to a less intensive but monitored medical ward. Patients who have undergone successful reperfusion, remain clinically stable, have no heart failure, have no recurrent myocardial ischemia, have an ejection fraction of >40%, and have no contraindication for a treadmill test are also at low risk. Alternatively, patients with recurrent ischemia by any measure, congestive heart failure, or high-grade arrhythmia are at high risk for death or further complications and may benefit from early cardiac catheterization.

Two groups of patients must be rapidly identified:

1. Patients in cardiogenic shock or who are developing cardiogenic shock
2. Patients who fail to reperfuse with thrombolytics

These patients should be urgently studied in the cath lab. In the case of cardiogenic shock, mortality can be substantially reduced by expeditious percutaneous coronary intervention (PCI). For patients who fail to reperfuse with thrombolytics, "rescue" angioplasty likely will be of benefit, though more data are needed to support this position. Although routine coronary angiography following thrombolytic therapy was demonstrated to be unhelpful in earlier studies, the situation may have changed with the introduction of aciximab and PCI. There is now a lower threshold to bring patients to the cath lab electively the day following AMI to define the anatomy and open the culprit artery with stenting. This is a very fluid area that is still evolving, and each CCU/cath lab team will likely develop its own strategies based on the most recent evidence.

Anterior and inferior/posterior MIs differ in a number of ways that result in differing prognoses for these two forms of infarction. Table 5-1 contrasts a number of features of anterior and inferior/posterior MI.

BIBLIOGRAPHY

Becker, R.C., Burns, M., Gore, J.M., et al. Early assessment and in-hospital management of patients with acute myocardial infarction at increased risk for adverse outcomes: A nationwide perspective of current clinical practice. *Am. Heart J.* 135:786–796, 1998.

Lamas, G.A., Mitchell, G.F., Flaker G.C., et al. Clinical significance of mitral regurgitation after acute myocardial infarction. *Circulation* 96:827–833, 1997.

Lee, L., Woodlief, L., Topol, E.J., et al. Predictors of 30-day mortality in the era of reperfusion for acute myocardial infarction: Results from an international trial of 41,021 patients. GUSTO-I Investigators. *Circulation* 91:1659–1668, 1995.

Mark, D.B., Sigmon, K., Topol, E.J., et al. Identification of acute myocardial infarction patients suitable for early hospital discharge after aggressive interventional therapy: Results from the Thrombolysis and Angioplasty in Acute Myocardial Infarction Registry. *Circulation* 83:1186–1193, 1991.

O'Connor, C.M., Hathaway, W.R., Bates, E.R., et al. Clinical characteristics and long-term outcome of patients in whom congestive heart failure develops after thrombolytic therapy for acute myocardial infarction: Development of a predictive model. *Am. Heart J.* 133:633–673, 1997.

Peterson, E.D., Shaw, L.J., and Califf, R.M. Guidelines for risk stratification after myocardial infarction. *Ann. Intern. Med.* 126:556–560, 1997.

Reeder, G.S. Identification and management of the low-risk patient after myocardial infarction. *ACC Curr. J. Rev.* May/June: 27–31, 1997.

6

The CCU Diet

Very little information is available to help guide the physician in selecting the best diet for a patient with an acute myocardial infarction (AMI).

Heavy meals can precipitate bouts of angina pectoris and are associated with an increase in myocardial oxygen consumption. Consequently, the coronary care unit (CCU) diet should be kept reasonably light: 1,200–1,500 cal/day.

Patients are generally not allowed to eat or drink, or are kept on fluids alone for a variable period of time (4–24 hours) after they first arrive in the CCU. This is done in order to observe them briefly, assuring the staff that the patients' vital signs and clinical state are relatively stable before they are allowed to eat. It is also necessary in case a patient needs an urgent procedure, such as angioplasty.

Meals may be served in small portions (six small feedings might be ideal) so as to diminish the possibility of increased postprandial cardiac output.

Many CCUs do not allow patients to ingest hot or cold fluids for fear that these may precipitate rhythm disturbances. Clinical studies do not support this prohibition for most patients, and it is now felt that patients may ingest hot or cold fluids if desired. In addition, many CCU diets prohibit the use of coffee or tea because of the fear that caffeine's sympathomimetic actions might cause arrhythmias. Patients may drink decaffeinated coffee or, if desired, weak tea, although no firm data exist to support the hypothesis that caffeine-containing beverages actually cause disturbances in rhythm.

Many patients admitted with MI have been eating a diet rich in saturated animal fats and high in cholesterol content. A great deal of evidence has implicated such a diet in causing atherosclerosis. Post MI patients should modify their diet by decreasing saturated fat and cholesterol intake (e.g., eggs, animal meat and fat, cream, butter) and increasing polyunsaturated fat intake (e.g., fish, chicken, vegetables, fruits). Consequently, a low-fat diet should be prescribed during the patient's entire hospitalization.

Decreased left ventricular function with a consequent decreased cardiac output can lead to sodium retention. Patients with MI should therefore not receive excessive amounts of sodium in their diet, since this can lead to hypervolemia and pulmonary congestion. On the other hand, severe sodium restriction can result in hypovolemia, accompanied by further depression of cardiac output, blood pressure, and urine flow. Thus, the no-added-salt diet (4–5 g NaCl in 24 hours) would seem to be a reasonable compromise.

Patients placed on bed rest and given drugs such as morphine and atropine (or drugs with atropine-like side effects) will frequently become constipated. Constipation results in straining at stool—the Valsalva maneuver—which has been shown to decrease coronary blood flow. To combat constipation, most patients are placed on stool-softening medication (e.g., dioctyl sodium sulfosuccinate) on arrival in the CCU. In addition, it seems reasonable to give average or even increased amounts of fiber in the diet of CCU patients to prevent constipation.

Some investigators feel strongly that glucose, insulin, and potassium solutions should be administered to patients with AMI (the polarizing solution of Sodi-Pallares). Conflicting evidence exists as to whether such treatment is efficacious in preventing arrhythmias and limiting infarct size (see Chapter 12). In the absence of conclusive evidence, it seems reasonable to include healthy amounts of glucose- and potassium-containing foods in the CCU diet. This is especially true for patients who receive potassium-wasting diuretics, whether or not they are receiving concomitant digitalis preparations.

In summary, a reasonable CCU diet is as follows:

PROTOCOL

1. Give nothing by mouth for the first 4–6 hours after the patient arrives in the CCU. Individualize initiation of feeding according to the patient's clinical status.
2. Offer a 1,200- to 1,500-cal, soft, bland, low-cholesterol and low-saturated-fat diet in six small feedings.
3. Include abundant glucose, potassium, and fiber, with approximately 4–5 g NaCl.

BIBLIOGRAPHY

Burch, G.E. Sick people's food. *Am. Heart J.* 85:279, 1973.

Cohen, I.M., Alpert, J.S., Francis, G.S., Vieweg, W.V.R., and Hagan, A.D. Safety of hot and cold liquids in patients with acute myocardial infarction. *Chest* 71:450–452, 1977.

Diaz, R., Paolasso, E.A., Piegas, L.S., Tajer, C.D., Moreno, M.G., Corvalan R., et al. Metabolic modulation of acute myocardial infarction—The ECLA glucose-insulin-potassium pilot trial. *Circulation* 98:2227–2234, 1998.

Eshleman, R. *American Heart Association Cookbook,* 4th ed. New York: Ballantine, 1988.

Houser, D. Ice water for MI patients? Why not? Another one of those traditions bites the dust. *Am. J. Nurs.* 76: 432–434, 1976.

Lader, E.W., and Kronzon, I. Ice-water-induced arrhythmias in a patient with ischemic heart disease. *Ann. Intern. Med.* 96:614–615, 1982.

Lynn, L.A., and Kissinger, J.F. Coronary precautions: Should caffeine be restricted in patients after myocardial infarction? *Heart Lung* 21:365–371, 1992.

Warren, S.E., Alpert, J.S., and Francis, G.S. Diet in the coronary care unit. *Am. Heart J.* 95:130–131, 1978.

7

Activity in the Hospital and Discharge from the Hospital

The risk of serious complications and death in patients with acute myocardial infarction (AMI) is highest during the first few hours and days after the onset of symptoms. The slight but definite risk that exists in the days following the acute event means that all patients with MI should remain in the hospital for a certain length of time. Past surveys of physicians treating patients with uncomplicated MI have shown that the median length of total hospital stay decreased from 21 days in 1970 to approximately 5 days currently. Ideally, a patient should be hospitalized only until the benefits of hospitalization no longer justify the expense. The only reasonable basis for deciding the appropriate discharge time is estimation of the risk of death and serious complications for the individual patient. Multivariate statistical techniques can be used to estimate individual patient risk, using various weighted variables to calculate the overall risk. Complications that tend to extend the hospital stay include heart failure, extension of MI, heart block, cardiac arrest, intraventricular conduction delay, and supraventricular tachycardia. Older patients have a higher mortality following AMI and require longer hospitalization. It is therefore important to tailor the hospital stay to the individual patient.

Current data suggest that most patients admitted to a coronary care unit (CCU) with a definite MI can be discharged from the hospital after 4–7 days. Most patients are transferred from the CCU to an intermediate cardiac care unit following 48–72 hours in the CCU. Such step-down units typically provide continued arrhythmia surveillance and have personnel who are skilled in the special needs of cardiac patients, including immediate resuscitation. Cardiac rehabilitation is usually initiated in this step-down or intermediate CCU.

Two protocols are suggested here. Various modifications can be made in these schedules, depending on the individual case, but experience indicates that the patient, house officers, and nurses all need some sort of definite guidelines concerning the patient's activity level following acute MI.

In general, discharge from the CCU and ambulation occur on schedule unless the patient develops chest pain, postural hypotension, severe fatigue, arrhythmias, marked tachycardia, or other complications. Other variables that must be considered in individualizing the amount of activity include the emotional and physical status of the patient before the attack, the patient's age, associated noncardiac problems, and the response of the patient to the management. Most patients should be allowed to sit in a comfortable chair on the first day after admission as long as they do not feel excessively fatigued. If complications do not occur, patients may gradually increase their activity and walk on day 3 of hospitalization. If conditions are appropriate, plans are made to go home on or about days 4–7. Patients increase their activity progressively to prepare for this. An accelerated 3- to 5-day admission protocol is also included at the end of this chapter, along with criteria for acceptance into this short-stay algorithm.

Before hospital discharge, most patients should perform a limited exercise test. The result of this test is predictive of subsequent mortality. Horizontal depression of the electrocardiographic (ECG) ST segment during exercise equal to or greater than 1 mm compared with the resting tracing or the precipitation of an episode of angina pectoris predicts greater morbidity or mortality for that patient during the first year after infarction. This has therapeutic implications and may warrant more aggressive treatment for these patients.

A limited exercise test with or without echocardiography or nuclear imaging following MI and before discharge is both safe and useful. Because of the low level of activity called for in the Naughton or modified Naughton (or modified Bruce) exercise protocol, the test allows patients to exert themselves much as they would at home. The physician immediately becomes aware of serious arrhythmias, a drop in systolic blood pressure, a low threshold for angina, or ST-segment depression—all or any of which might alter therapy or possibly indicate further diagnostic steps such as coronary angiography. The exercise test is often not performed on elderly or incapacitated patients—e.g., those with overt heart failure, those who have had recent rest angina, those with a physical handicap that precludes exercise, and those who refuse informed consent. It is expected that most patients will perform favorably during exercise, which then offers added psychological comfort to both physician and patient. Exercise testing provides the basis for rational and individualized guidelines for physical activity following discharge. For example, if the patient achieves a maximal heart rate of 120 beats per minute and a peak systolic blood pressure of 165 mm Hg during limited exercise testing with no untoward results, it is likely that sexual activity may be resumed soon after discharge. Most adult males achieve a heart rate of less than 120 beats per minute and a peak systolic blood pressure of less than 165 mm Hg during sexual intercourse with a spouse (see Chapter 33). Other ordinary physical activities may also be more logically advised following successful completion of the exercise test.

Patients whose hospital course has been complicated by heart failure, shock, persistent high-grade ventricular ectopy or cardiac arrest, recurrent angina, or infarct extension require special consideration. Holter monitoring and radionuclide ventriculography or echocardiography can identify a high-risk subgroup of patients who have persistent high-grade ventricular arrhythmias and/or low ejection fraction. Signal-averaged ECG and/or electrophysiologic testing may be indicated in such patients.

Patients with evidence of residual ischemia by provocative testing or with episodes of post-infarct angina should undergo cardiac catheterization prior to discharge to determine whether they are candidates for either elective coronary artery bypass grafting or angioplasty. The physician's final diagnostic and therapeutic recommendations should continue to be individually tailored for each institution and each patient.

PROTOCOL FOR A 4- TO 7-DAY ADMISSION

Days 1–2 Bed rest in the CCU; the patient may be up in a chair on the day of admission if stable and if tolerated.

Days 3–4 Moderate activity in the intermediate cardiac unit. The patient may use a chair most of the day and a bedside commode and may be walking by day 3–4.

Days 4–7 Increasing activity—i.e., walking in the corridor is allowed. The patient may shower and wash hair; may undergo a limited exercise test on days 4–7, prior to discharge.

PROTOCOL FOR A 3- TO 5-DAY ADMISSION

1. Patients eligible for a 3- to 5-day admission are individuals with typical symptoms of AMI combined with ECG and enzyme criteria for the diagnosis of AMI who, 48 hours after admission, have evidenced *none* of the following:

- angina
- congestive heart failure (rales and/or an S_3)
- systolic blood pressure less than 90 mm Hg
- left ventricular ejection fraction less than 35% (if known)
- ventricular arrhythmias of Lown class 2 or more (multifocal pre-ventricular contractions or more advanced ectopy)
- second- or third-degree heart block
- psychological or intellectual incapacity to cooperate with medical personnel.

2. Many but not all of these individuals will have received pharmacologic thrombolytic therapy. Some will have undergone cardiac catheterization with or without percutaneous transluminal coronary angioplasty (PTCA).

3. Patients discharged in 3–5 days must have a home situation that is concordant with performance of the protocol (i.e., a family member or friend must live with the patient and be prepared to drive the patient to the hospital for cardiac rehabilitation sessions).

4. Patients who undergo cardiac catheterization should have a left ventricular ejection fraction greater than 35% and coronary arterial anatomy deemed "stable" by the attending cardiologist. Example: A 60-year-old patient with an old inferior MI and a totally occluded right coronary artery presents with a new anterior MI. The patient is treated with intravenous thrombolytic therapy and subsequent cardiac catheterization demonstrates a 50% stenosis in the left anterior descending coronary artery and the previously described 100% blocked right coronary artery. This patient's coronary anatomy is deemed stable. PTCA or a coronary artery bypass graft operation is not necessarily indicated.

5. All patients undergo an exercise test on either the third, fourth, or fifth hospital day. Individuals with minimal or no ischemia are eligible for early discharge.

6. Patients must give informed consent for early discharge. Oral consent is satisfactory.

7. Patients eligible for early discharge receive an accelerated educational and exercise program during their inpatient stay. The exact nature of this protocol is determined by the nursing and cardiac rehabilitation staff.

8. Patients are eligible for the early discharge program even if they spend their entire hospitalization in the CCU.

9. Following discharge from the hospital, patients return for an outpatient cardiac rehabilitation program. Patients participate in this program until the rehabilitation nurse or technician is satisfied with the patient's clinical status and knowledge acquisition.

BIBLIOGRAPHY

Abraham, A.S., Sever, Y., Weinstein, M., Dollberg, M., and Menczel, J. Value of early ambulation in patients with and without complications after acute myocardial infarction. *N. Engl. J. Med.* 292:719–722, 1975.

Hamm, L.F., Stull, G.H., and Crow, R.S. Exercise testing early after myocardial infarction: Historic perspective and current uses. *Prog. Cardiovasc. Dis.* 28:463–476, 1986.

Madsen, E.B., Hougaard, P., Gilpin, E., and Pedersen, A. The length of hospitalization after acute myocardial infarction determined by risk calculation. *Circulation* 68:9–16, 1983.

Mark, D.B., Sigmon, K., Topol, E.J., et al. Identification of acute myocardial infarction patients suitable for early hospital discharge after aggressive therapy. *Circulation* 83:1186–1193, 1991.

Rowe, M.H., Jelinek, M.V., Liddell, N., Hugens, M. Effect of rapid mobilization on ejection fractions and ventricular volumes after acute myocardial infarction. *Am. J. Cardiol.* 63:1037–1041, 1989.

Theroux, P., Waters, D.D., Halphen, C., Debaisieux, J.C., and Mizgala, H.F. Prognostic value of exercise testing soon after myocardial infarction. *N. Engl. J. Med.* 301: 341–345, 1979.

Topol, E.J., Burek, K., O'Neill, W.W., et al. A randomized controlled trial of hospital discharge three days after myocardial infarction in the era of reperfusion. *N. Engl. J. Med.* 318:1083–1088, 1988.

8

Suggested Orders in Suspected or Routine Myocardial Infarction

Many different therapeutic regimens are employed in the management of patients with acute myocardial infarction (AMI). Probably most of these programs are successful. The following set of orders constitutes a suggested program for a patient admitted to the coronary care unit (CCU) with a suspected MI. The orders themselves are written in capital letters, and the comment that follows explains the purpose of that particular order.

1. ADMIT TO CCU WITH THE DIAGNOSIS OF SUSPECTED MI.

   Some hospitals prefer the diagnosis to be MI or unstable angina/possible MI. The diagnosis of MI is discussed in Chapter 11.

2. STATUS: CRITICAL.

   This is an administrative order, which warns of the potential seriousness of the patient's condition (see Chapter 2).

3. BED CHAIR ACTIVITY WITH COMMODE PRIVILEGES ONCE PATIENT IS STABLE.

   Strict bed rest is probably not good for patients with acute MI. It can result in atrophy of normal baroreceptor function, so that the patient has problems with orthostatic hypotension when he or she is beginning to walk. Consequently, short periods of sitting up in a chair (e.g., 20 minutes b.i.d.) may be allowed right from the first day of hospitalization if the patient is stable. Patients with cardiogenic shock or severe left ventricular failure are usually not candidates for this form of early mobilization. Patients are frequently more comfortable and less disturbed if allowed to use a bedside commode or even a nearby toilet instead of a bedpan. Activity is discussed in Chapter 7.

4. VITAL SIGNS Q30MIN × 4; Q60MIN × 2; IF STABLE, Q2–4H THROUGH THE FIRST 24 HOURS: Q4–6H THEREAFTER.

   The frequency of recording vital signs varies from hospital to hospital. Temperature need be taken only b.i.d.

Thus, most of the time, vital signs consist of respiratory rate, blood pressure, and pulse.

5. DIET: 1,500 CAL, LOW CHOLESTEROL, LOW SATURATED FAT; INCREASED BULK, GLUCOSE, AND POTASSIUM; NO ADDED SALT.

Diet is discussed in Chapter 6.

6. ORAL FLUID INTAKE RESTRICTED TO 1,000 ML PER 8-HOUR PERIOD.

This works out to approximately 2,000 ml/day because patients have little intake during the night, when they are asleep. Older CCU regimens restricted fluids stringently, but hemodynamic data have demonstrated that most patients without overt left ventricular failure are not volume-overloaded and should have a moderate fluid intake.

7. OXYGEN SUPPLEMENTATION BY NASAL PRONGS (2 L/min or more as required).

Oxygen therapy is discussed in Chapter 10. Many cardiologists encourage their patients to take a deep breath q20min while awake.

8. ELECTROCARDIOGRAM (ECG) Q8H × 3.

Patients with complications usually require additional ECGs.

9. PORTABLE CHEST RADIOGRAPHY ON ADMISSION.

This is obtained to monitor pulmonary congestion secondary to left ventricular failure. Patients should be sitting up when the radiograph is obtained. If the chest x-ray is unremarkable, further chest roentgenograms are not necessary unless heart failure is suspected.

10. LABORATORY WORK

a. SERUM MARKERS OF MYOCARDIAL NECROSIS: Q8H × 3.

Various combinations of creatine kinase (CK, CKMB), troponin, and myoglobin are obtained. CKMB and/or troponin determinations are usually ordered on admission and q8–12h for a total of three samples during the first 24–36 hours of hospitalization. (See Chapter 11 for a discussion of the diagnostic use of serum markers of myocardial necrosis in MI.)

b. ELECTROLYTE DETERMINATIONS: QD × 2–3 DAYS.

A knowledge of serum Na and K is particularly important in patients who are receiving diuretics and digitalis preparations. Moreover, changes in cardiac output, intravenous infusion rates, and diet can all influence serum electrolytes. Since electrolytes can have a major effect on cell excitability and since patients with MI are already prone to arrhythmias secondary to altered cell excitability, it is vital to follow serum electrolytes until the patient's condition is stable. Patients whose courses are stable and who are not receiving diuretics do not need daily determination of serum electrolytes.

c. OTHER BLOOD TESTS: CREATININE, GLUCOSE, BUN, TOTAL PROTEIN, ALBUMIN, CALCIUM, MAGNESIUM, PHOSPHORUS, CHOLESTEROL, HEMATOCRIT, WBC, PROTHROMBIN TIME (PROTIME) and C-reactive protein.

The C-reactive protein may have important independent prognostic information and should be ordered on admission. Periodic determinations of serum creatinine, glucose (daily or more often in diabetics), BUN, total protein, albumin, calcium, and phosphorus all aid in the management of acutely ill patients. These determinations need not be made more than once in relatively stable patients. In most patients they are obtained only on admission. Serum lipids frequently demonstrate an early fall with MI. However, values obtained early during the first day of hospitalization tell the physician whether the patient is usually hyperlipidemic. A daily hematocrit is required for patients with acute MI, since there can be a fall in this measurement during the patient's first few days in the hospital. This fall is probably related to frequent bloodletting. An occasional patient has an increase in hematocrit. The latter finding usually implies significant dehydration. Some CCUs follow WBCs and erythrocyte sedimentation rates following MI. Both measurements show moderate elevations early in the course of acute MI, and they remain elevated for approximately 1–2 weeks after MI (see Chapter 11). Persistently elevated values are often a sign of Dressler's syndrome (late autoimmune pericarditis), discussed in Chapter 20. A rough screen of coagulation is obtained with a protime. In a rare patient—particularly one in shock or with severe left ventricular failure—disseminated intravascular coagulation may develop and require frequent protimes as well as other tests of the integrity of the coagulation cascade. Protime and partial thromboplastin time are followed carefully in patients receiving warfarin and heparin, respectively (see Chapters 13 and 14). The average stable patient needs to have a protime determined only on admission if this value is normal.

11. DAILY WEIGHTS AND INTAKE AND OUTPUT.
    The recording of daily weights and of intake and output is particularly important in patients with left ventricular failure.

12. INTRAVENOUS INFUSION OF 5% D/W HELD AT A LOW INFUSION RATE.
    A central venous pressure line or shorter plastic cannula is the preferred type of intravenous line. Scalpvein needles are too easily dislodged and hence may become infiltrated at a critical moment.

13. MEDICATIONS
    a. LAXATIVES, STOOL SOFTENERS, OR BOTH.
        Generally, a daily stool softener is ordered to prevent straining at stool. (See the discussion of increased fiber in the diet and its combination with stool-softening medication in Chapter 6.) Patients who are constipated despite stool softeners should be given a gentle laxative such as milk of magnesia (usually administered h.s.).
    b. TRANQUILIZERS.
        Psychological factors play an important role in the genesis of arrhythmias (see Chapter 2). A mild sedative is usually prescribed for patients with acute MI. The usual choice is one of several benzodiazepines, e.g., alprazolam (0.25 mg) t.i.d. or q.i.d. A sleeping medication is also frequently required, because patients with acute MI experience anxiety-related difficulties in falling asleep. Flurazepam (30 mg) is often employed, since it tends not to disturb REM sleep patterns.
    c. ANALGESICS.
        Acetaminophen is usually effective for minor discomfort, while morphine, hydromorphone (Dilaudid), or meperidine (Demerol) is usually required for initial control of the pain of MI. Repeated doses of analgesics should be given q10–15min until pain is relieved (see Chapter 9).

    d. ANTICOAGULANTS.

It has been clearly demonstrated that small subcutaneous doses of heparin administered q8–12h prevent thrombophlebitis and associated pulmonary embolism in patients with MI. Early ambulation schedules also reduce this complication and make "minidose" heparin, if employed, necessary for only a few days (see Chapter 14). Some cardiologists recommend the use of warfarin anticoagulants routinely in patients with MI. This is a highly controversial subject (see Chapter 14). For a discussion of the use of thrombolytic agents in patients with hyperacute MI, see Chapter 13.

PROTOCOL

1. Admit the patient to the CCU with the diagnosis MI.
2. Status: critical.
3. Activity: bed and chair with commode privileges for 12–24 hours.
4. Vital signs: q30min × 4; q60min × 2; if stable, q4–6h through first 24 hours and then q6h thereafter.
5. Diet: NPO until stable (4–24 hours); thereafter 1,500 cal, low cholesterol, no-added-salt diet (see Chapter 6).
6. Oral fluids restricted to 1,000 ml/8 h.
7. Oxygen at 2 L/min by nasal prongs.
8. ECG q8h × 3.
9. Upright portable chest radiograph on admission and as needed thereafter.
10. Blood work: CKMB (three determinations during the first 24 hours) and/or troponin q8h × 3. Na, K, Cl, CO_2, CBC, BUN, glucose, creatinine on admission and as often as indicated (every day, every other day, or less frequently) thereafter. On admission only: total protein, albumin, calcium, magnesium, phosphorus, cholesterol.
11. Daily weights and intake/output.
12. IV: keep open with 5% D/W.
13. Medications:
    a. Dioctyl sodium sulfosuccinate, 100 mg PO qd; milk of magnesia, 30 ml PO hs PRN for constipation.
    b. Alprazolam, 0.25 mg (1 tab) PO q6h.
    c. Aspirin, 325 mg PO qd. Morphine, 5 mg, hydromorphone (Dilaudid), 2 mg, or meperidine, 50 mg (dosage is variable depending on patient's size, sensitivity to narcotics, severity of pain, relative con-

traindications) IV PRN for severe pain (usually administered by a nurse using a strict protocol). Repeat doses should be given q10–15min until pain is relieved (see Chapter 9 for a complete discussion of pain relief in AMI).

14. For thrombolytic therapy, see Chapter 13.
15. For therapy of specific complications, see Chapters 17–26.

BIBLIOGRAPHY

Herlitz, J. Analgesia in myocardial infarction. *Drugs* 37: 939–944, 1989.

Lagrand, W.K., Visser, C.A., Hermens, W.T., Niessen, H.W.M., Verheugt, F.W.A., Wolbink, G-J, and Hack, C.E. C-reactive protein as a cardiovascular risk factor: More than an epiphenomenon? *Circulation* 100: 96–102, 1999.

Ryan, T.J., Anderson, J.L., Antman, E.M., Braniff, B.A., Brooks, N.H., Califf, R.M., et al. ACC/AHA Guidelines for the management of patients with acute myocardial infarction. *J. Am. Coll. Cardiol.* 28:1328–1428, 1996.

9

Control of Pain after Acute Myocardial Infarction

Control of pain or discomfort is a key goal in the management of patients with acute myocardial infarction (AMI). A vicious cycle is set up whereby pain begets anxiety, which activates the sympathetic nervous system, thereby driving heightened myocardial oxygen demand and further myocardial ischemia, leading to more pain (Fig. 9-1). Patients with AMI are usually well aware of their tenuous situation, are often extremely anxious, and are truly in need of physician interaction. Prompt control of discomfort initiates a welcome partnership between patient and physician.

The root of chest discomfort in the setting of AMI is myocardial ischemia. Acute aortic dissection, pericarditis, and pulmonary infarction should always be considered as alternative diagnoses, as they have very different management strategies. The treatment of chest discomfort emanating from AMI is the treatment of severe myocardial ischemia and infarction. Coronary reperfusion, intravenous beta-adrenergic blockade, intravenous nitroglycerin (NTG), and analgesics such as morphine sulfate are indicated. Supportive reassurance and psychological support by the physician are also necessary.

Although once considered contraindicated, sub-lingual (SL) NTG is now commonly given to patients with AMI, often in the emergency room. Intravenous nitroglycerin should be started promptly (unless the patient is hypotensive or has clear evidence of a right ventricular infarct), so as not to allow the systolic blood pressure to go below 100 mm Hg. A typical early dose of intravenous nitroglycerin might be 30–60 µg/min. If titration to very high doses is necessary, nitrate tolerance is probably occurring. Nitrates both reduce left ventricular filling pressure, thereby reducing wall stress (a major component of myocardial oxygen demand), and improve coronary blood flow. Though not demonstrated to improve mortality in AMI, nitrates clearly relieve chest discomfort and pulmonary vascular congestion; they should therefore be part of the routine management of an uncomplicated MI. Rarely, hypotension and severe bradycardia can occur with intravenous nitroglycerin, the result of activation of ventricular mechanoreceptors (the Bezold-Jarisch reflex). When this occurs, lying the patient

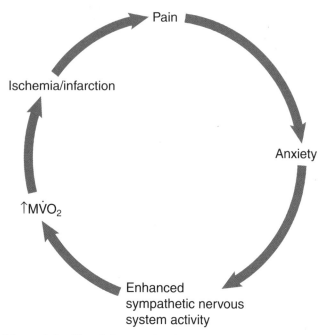

Figure 9-1. The vicious cycle of pain in acute myocardial infarction. MV̇O₂, myocardial oxygen consumption.

down and raising the legs, along with volume expansion of the circulation, is usually sufficient to restore blood pressure and heart rate.

Thrombolytic therapy or percutaneous coronary intervention with reperfusion is the most powerful tool to reduce chest discomfort. In fact, if thrombolytic therapy does not alleviate chest pain, failure of reperfusion should be considered and "rescue" angioplasty may be necessary.

Intravenous beta-adrenergic blockers, such as four metoprolol, should be given unless contraindicated (i.e., cardiogenic shock, severe heart failure, advanced A-V heart block, bradycardia, severe chronic obstructive lung disease, or severe asthma). The dose of four metoprolol is highly variable and should be titrated to slow heart rate to less than 70 beats per minute and to control blood pressure (Chapter 15). It is customary to start with 10–15 mg of metoprolol given slowly intravenously and switch to oral therapy (50–100 mg b.i.d.) when the patient has stabilized. Intravenous beta-adrenergic blockers frequently help to reduce the pain of

AMI. About 80% of patients with AMI can safely be given beta blockers.

Morphine sulfate is a time-honored treatment for the pain and anxiety of AMI. The dose should be titrated, but a total dose of 7–15 mg is usually sufficient. Occasionally, very large doses up to 25 mg are necessary to control pain. A dose of 3–5 mg may be repeated at 10- to 15-minute intervals as needed. Morphine SO_4 reduces left ventricular filling pressure, lowers blood pressure and heart rate, attenuates sympathetic activity, and greatly reduces anxiety and breathlessness. Symptomatic hypotension occurs in 2–3% of patients following the use of morphine SO_4 and can occur in both anterior and inferior AMI. In response to hypotension, the heart rate may be inappropriately decreased due to parasympathetic nervous system augmentation. Nausea occurs in 20–30% of patients given morphine sulfate, and 5–15% of patients have emesis. About 1% will develop respiratory failure.

In general, the chest discomfort of patients with AMI should be treated first with anti-ischemic therapy, including thrombolytics or percutaneous coronary intervention, nitrates, and beta-adrenergic blockers. Small doses of morphine sulfate may be necessary to help alleviate excessive pain, anxiety, and the hyper-adrenergic state. Persistence of severe pain after treatment with thrombolytic therapy, nitrates, and beta-adrenergic blockers is a poor prognostic sign and may require urgent catheterization (rescue angioplasty) to open the culprit artery.

PROTOCOL

1. Reassurance and psychological support should be given to all patients to decrease anxiety and agitation.
   Hypotension can occur following nitroglycerin, especially in patients with right ventricular or acute inferior MIs. Careful monitoring of blood pressure is necessary when using NTG in the setting of AMI. Hypotension is treated by placing the patient in a reverse Trendelenburg (head-down) position and administering IV fluids.

2. Patients with presumptive MI should receive aspirin (324 mg) and SL NTG (0.3 or 0.4 mg). A second and subsequently a third SL NTG may be administered at 5-minute intervals.

3. IV beta blocker (metoprolol 10–15 mg) should be given unless contraindicated. Titrate as needed to control heart rate and blood pressure. The dose is highly variable.

4. Reperfusion therapy as soon as possible when not con-traindicated.
5. Morphine sulfate 3–5 mg repeated at 10- to 15-minute intervals to a maximal dose of 7–15 mg.
6. Patients with severe, unrelenting pain despite all ther-apy should be considered for urgent cardiac catheteriza-tion and percutaneous coronary intervention.

BIBLIOGRAPHY

Alderman, E.L. Analgesics in the acute phase of myocardial infarction. *J.A.M.A.* 229: 1646–1648, 1974.

Come, P.C., and Pitt, B. Nitroglycerin-induced severe hypo-tension and bradycardia in patients with acute myocar-dial infarction. *Circulation* 54: 624–628, 1976.

Herlitz, J., Hjalmarson, Å., Holmberg, S., et al. Variability, prediction and prognostic significance of chest pain in acute myocardial infarction. *Cardiology* 73: 13–21, 1986.

Herlitz, J., Hjalmarson, Å., Waagstein, F. Beta blockade and chest pain in acute myocardial infarction. *Am. Heart J.* 112: 1120–1126, 1986.

Lee, G., DeMaria, A.N., Amsterdam, E.A., et al. Compara-tive effects of morphine, meperidine, and pentazocine on cardiocirculatory dynamics in patients with acute myocar-dial infarction. *Am. J. Med.* 60: 949–955, 1976.

Lee, G., Low, R.I., Amsterdam, E.A., et al. Hemodynamic effects of morphine and nalbuphine in acute myocardial infarction. *Clin. Pharmacol. Ther.* 29: 576–581, 1981.

10

Arterial Blood Gases and Supplemental Oxygen Therapy

Patients with acute myocardial infarction (AMI) are commonly hypoxemic, especially when left ventricular failure or cardiogenic shock is present. Various pathophysiologic mechanisms have been proposed to explain this finding, including (a) ventilation/perfusion imbalances in the lungs, (b) collapse of small airways with resultant right-to-left shunting, and (c) interstitial and alveolar pulmonary edema. A number of studies suggest that a component of the pulmonary extravascular fluid collection that often occurs after MI may not be due solely to elevation in pulmonary microvascular pressure; altered capillary permeability may also play a role. Oxygen inhalation therapy has been in widespread use for patients with acute MI for many years. At least one controlled study (Rawles and Kenmore, 1976) was unable to document any difference in mortality rate or arrhythmias in patients with AMI receiving oxygen therapy, but it is considered conventional therapy in all hospitals. Oxygen therapy does result in a modest systemic vasoconstriction and in a slight decrease in cardiac output. These changes, however, are usually of no clinical consequence, and it seems reasonable to correct the frequently present modest hypoxemia.

Low-flow oxygen should be administered to most patients with AMI, usually in the range of 2 to 5 L/min by nasal cannula. Patients with congestive heart failure or shock may benefit from higher concentrations (40% to 100% oxygen), whereas patients with severe obstructive lung disease and carbon dioxide retention may require much less (1 to 2 L/min) or none at all. Worsening hypoxemia can be due to atelectasis, pneumonia, pulmonary embolism, or heart failure. Arterial blood gases should be drawn as necessary to assess the patient's condition and response to therapy.

PROTOCOL

1. Patients should be placed on supplemental oxygen, 2 L/min by nasal prongs, on arrival in the CCU.
2. Arterial blood gases should be determined approximately 5 to 10 minutes after the initiation of oxygen therapy.

A convenient technique for obtaining arterial blood that produces minimal discomfort is radial artery puncture with a 22-gauge needle through a small intraepidermal wheal of 1% lidocaine. Be sure that the inside of the syringe is thoroughly coated with heparin and that heparin fills the dead space of the syringe and needle. The latter maneuver prevents air bubbles from getting in contact with the arterial blood sample.

3. If the P_{O_2} in the arterial blood sample is less than 80 mm Hg, the delivery of supplemental O_2 should be increased to 4 L/min and repeat arterial blood gases obtained 5 to 10 minutes later.

4. If the arterial P_{O_2} is still less than 80 mm Hg, supplemental oxygen should be delivered by face mask rather than nasal prongs. In severely hypoxemic patients, such as those with pulmonary edema, oxygen supplementation should be initiated by the face-mask route. Intubation may sometimes be necessary or, for some patients, non-invasive ventilatory support may suffice.

5. Failure to obtain adequate arterial P_{O_2} values with face-mask oxygen delivery should result in a switch to a rebreathing face mask apparatus for oxygen supplementation.

6. Oxygen therapy should be continued at least as long as the patient is in the CCU and probably until the patient is ambulatory with no demonstrable hypoxemia.

7. If pulmonary embolism is suspected, it may be helpful to obtain arterial blood gases while the patient is breathing room air. Oxygen therapy need be discontinued for only 7 minutes in patients without pulmonary disease in order to obtain a blood sample representative of room-air pulmonary function. If the patient has clinically significant obstructive pulmonary disease, it is necessary to withhold oxygen for 25 minutes before the arterial blood sample is obtained.

BIBLIOGRAPHY

Antonelli, M., Conti G., Rocco, M., et al. A comparison of non-invasive positive-pressure ventilation and conventional mechanical ventilation in patients with acute respiratory failure. *N. Engl. J. Med.* 339:429–435, 1998.

Biddle, T.L., Yu, P.N., Hodges, M., et al. Hypoxemia and lung water in acute myocardial infarction. *Am. Heart J.* 92:692–699, 1976.

Fillmore, S.J., Guimaraes, A.C., Scheidt, S.S., and Killip, T. Blood-gas changes and pulmonary hemodynamics following acute myocardial infarction. *Circulation* 45:583–591, 1971.

Gray, B.A., Hyde, R.W., Hodges, M., and Yu, P.N. Alterations in lung volume and pulmonary function in relation to hemodynamic changes in acute myocardial infarction. *Circulation* 59:551–559, 1979.

Hillberg, R.E., Johnson, D.C. Noninvasive ventilation. *N. Engl. J. Med.* 337: 1746–1752, 1997.

Loeb, H.S., Chuquimia, R., Sinno, M.Z., Rhaimtoola, S.H., Rosen, K.M., and Gunnar, R.M. Effects of low-flow oxygen on the hemodynamics and left ventricular function in patients with uncomplicated acute myocardial infarction. *Chest* 60:352–355, 1971.

Madias JE, and Hood WB, Jr. Reduction of precordial ST segment elevation in patients with acute myocardial infarction by oxygen breathing. *Circulation* 53 (suppl. I): 198–200, 1976.

Radvany, P., Maroko, P.R., and Braunwald, E. Effects of hypoxemia on the extent of myocardial necrosis after experimental coronary occlusion. *Am J. Cardiol.* 35: 795–800, 1975.

Raffin, T.A. Indications for arterial blood gas analysis. *Ann. Intern. Med.* 105:390–398, 1986.

Rawles, J., and Kenmore, A.C.F. Controlled trial of oxygen therapy in uncomplicated myocardial infarction. *Br. Med. J.* 1:1121–1123, 1976.

Sukumalchantra, Y., Danzig, R., Levy, S.E., and Swan, H.J.C. The mechanism of arterial hypoxemia in acute myocardial infarction. *Circulation* 41:641–650, 1970.

Thomas, M., Malmcrona, R., and Shillingford, J. Hemodynamic effects of oxygen in patients with acute myocardial infarction. *Br. Heart J.* 27:401–407, 1965.

11

ECG, Serum Markers, Serial Chest Radiographic Changes, Myocardial Imaging, Radionuclide Ventriculography, and Echocardiography

ELECTROCARDIOGRAM

Standard textbooks should be consulted by medical personnel charged with the care of patients with acute myocardial infarction (AMI). The initial electrocardiogram (ECG) should be studied carefully and repeated if there is any change in the patient's clinical condition. The rhythm, rate, and time of the tracing should be recorded on the chart along with the diagnosis. The initial ECG allows for early risk stratification and is critical in determining the optimal treatment strategy. Patients presenting after 20 minutes but within 6 hours of the onset of chest pain accompanied by ECG signs of 0.1 mV, or greater ST-segment elevation in two or more limb leads or 0.2 mV or greater elevation in two or more contiguous precordial leads, should be considered for prompt thrombolytic treatment or primary angioplasty unless there is a contraindication. In the Global Utilization of Streptokinase and T-PA for Occluded Coronary Arteries (GUSTO-1) trial, 34,166 of 41,021 patients who presented within 6 hours of chest pain with ST-segment elevation and no confounding factors—such as paced rhythms, ventricular rhythms, or left bundle-branch block (LBBB)—had their ECGs carefully analyzed prior to thrombolysis. In this patient cohort, the sum of ST-segment deviation, heart rate, QRS duration (for anterior infarct), and ECG evidence for previous infarction were significant predictors of 30-day mortality. Increased T-wave amplitude is one of the earliest ECG changes following coronary artery occlusion. Higher T waves in the presenting ECG probably represent earlier time to treatment and are associated with a lower mortality following thrombolytic therapy.

About 10% of patients presenting to the hospital with possible AMI have LBBB on the ECG. However, the timely availability of a previous ECG is the exception. The presence of LBBB on the presenting ECG may conceal the changes of

45

AMI, which can delay recognition and treatment. Patients with new LBBB should be considered to have AMI in the setting of prolonged chest discomfort. A new LBBB in patients with AMI correlates with occlusion of the proximal left anterior descending coronary artery, a large amount of jeopardized myocardium, and a higher rate of complications and death. Three ECG criteria aid in the diagnosis of AMI in patients with LBBB:

1. ST-segment elevation of 1 mm or more in the same direction as the QRS complex
2. ST-segment depression of 1 mm or more in lead V_1, V_2, or V_3
3. ST-segment elevation of 5 mm or more that is discordant (in the opposite direction from) with the QRS

The evidence favors an aggressive approach to the patient with discomfort due to acute myocardial ischemia and LBBB, as there is much to gain by giving thrombolytic therapy.

Transmural infarctions with ST-T elevation, or Q-wave infarctions, are characterized by the evolution of Q waves. Non-transmural infarctions, also known as non-Q-wave infarctions or sub-endocardial infarctions, are characterized by ST-segment and T-wave changes; they may involve sizable amounts of myocardium, or they may be small. The distinction between "transmural" and "non-transmural" infarction is somewhat arbitrary, and the terminology is confusing. About half of all autopsy proven sub-endocardial (i.e., non-Q-wave) infarcts are accompanied by Q waves, while half of transmural infarcts are not. However, patients with transmural or Q-wave infarction may have more early complications and higher early mortality, whereas those with non-transmural or non-Q-wave infarction have more early recurrent myocardial ischemia and re-infarction. Overall, the post-MI course of the two categories is essentially identical. It is recognized by some that non-Q-wave infarction is often an "incomplete" infarction, and aggressive (early) use of coronary angiography is often recommended. Although this strategy has recently been challenged, diagnostic catheterization is often performed in patients with non-Q-wave myocardial infarction, as recurrent myocardial ischemia is frequent and guidelines for thrombolytic reperfusion do not apply. Use of the terms *ST-T-wave–elevation infarct* and *non-ST-T-wave–elevation infarct* is more in keeping with modern thrombolytic strategies.

SERUM MARKERS FOR
ACUTE MYOCARDIAL INFARCTION

Since the mid-1970s, creatine kinase-MB (CK-MB) has served as the "gold standard" among biochemical markers of AMI. Creatine kinase is a high-energy-transfer cytoplasmic enzyme that is released when there is anoxic death of the cell. CK-MB is increased within 2 to 3 hours of AMI, and peak enzyme levels are reached 8 to 10 hours after the onset of chest pain. Sequential CK-MB levels are usually taken on admission and 12 and 24 hours later. A CK-MB level twice normal is generally considered to be the threshold for acute MI. The phenomenon of isolated elevations of CK-MB with normal CK occasionally occurs. The elevation of CK may be missed or may be misinterpreted if the entire rise and fall is within the normal range, especially if the baseline value of CK is low. Such patients are believed to have suffered a small infarction and have a good prognosis.

The CK-MB isoenzyme is relatively specific for myocardial damage, and generally the CK-MB parallels that of the total CK. The CK-MB may peak earlier than the total CK and may decline more rapidly. Patients who reperfuse with thrombolysis or primary angioplasty tend to have an earlier and higher peak CK-MB level if the occluded artery is successfully opened, presumably related to "washout" of the enzymes by reperfusion.

Skeletal muscle damage can result in detectable levels of CK-MB in the plasma. However, small amounts of damage to healthy skeletal muscle do not usually release enough CK-MB into plasma to cause diagnostic confusion. Patients with severe hypothyroidism have increased CK-MB levels due to skeletal myopathy and a decreased rate of clearance. Small increases in CK-MB are sometimes seen after angioplasty and/or stent deployment. Although a contentious issue, these small "bumps" in CK-MB following percutaneous coronary intervention may represent small amounts of myocardial necrosis from micro-emboli, and such patients are at greater risk for future coronary events.

The ratio of CK-MB to total CK has been proposed as helpful in the diagnosis of acute MI. A CK-MB level of 5% or more of the total CK has a sensitivity of 34% and a specificity of 88%. However, when high levels of CK are released due to skeletal muscle injury, a large amount of CK-MB must be released from the myocardium to meet these 5% criteria, which decreases the sensitivity of this method even further.

Patients with a rising and falling pattern of CK-MB and a peak value that exceeds the upper limit of the reference range should be considered to have an AMI regardless of CK-MB/total CK ratio.

Infarct size can be estimated after acute MI if several factors are known:

1. The amount of marker lost from the myocardium
2. The volume of distribution of the marker
3. The release ratio of the marker

The calculations can be difficult because disappearance rates are often unknown, about 85% of CK-MB is deactivated in lymph, and regional blood flow and washout from thrombolysis are variable. Nevertheless, large increases in CK and CK-MB are considered to be associated with substantial myocardial necrosis. There is less information regarding troponins and infarct size.

TROPONIN

Troponin T, I, and C are proteins that regulate calcium-dependent interactions between myosin and actin. The isoforms of troponin are tissue-specific and are the products of different genes. Peak troponin levels typically occur at 14 hours and again at 3 to 5 days following the index event, reflecting a biphasic pattern of protein release. Troponin levels, like those of CK, increase markedly and peak earlier following successful thrombolysis. A rapid-access "point of care" bedside kit for troponin T has recently become available, which might prove useful in the triage of low-risk patients away from or out of the CCU.

Most laboratories continue to use CK and CK-MB as the diagnostic tests of choice for the diagnosis of AMI. However, this is gradually changing as more experience is gained with troponins. Cardiac troponin appears within 3 hours of AMI symptoms, is more specific for cardiac tissue than CK-MB, and continues to be released up to 11 days after the index event, allowing for diagnosis in patients admitted late in the course of AMI. These advantages of troponin are increasingly recognized by hospital laboratories, many of which now offer both CK and troponin blood levels.

Several large clinical trials, including GUSTO, have indicated that troponin-T levels >0.1 µg/ml are associated with a higher 30-day mortality even after adjusting for ECG and CK-MB findings. Patients with unstable angina and normal CK and CK-MB values with slightly elevated troponin-T levels are at greater risk for future coronary events and hospital admission. Recognition of this fact has made the distinction between MI and unstable angina less clear. It is likely, though not proven, that small incremental changes in troponin represent micro-necrosis. Patients with unstable angina or non-Q-wave MI and cardiac troponin I levels >0.4 µg/ml also have a significantly increased 6-week mortality. Both troponin I and troponin T have independent prognostic power in patients with unstable angina and AMI. The two troponin markers are equally sensitive and have rather similar specificities. Because of our ability to detect very small amounts of myocardial damage with troponins, we are now finding more and more patients who have biochemical evidence for necrosis but do not meet criteria by conventional CK and CK-MB standards for AMI. It is increasingly more difficult to distinguish small MIs from unstable angina in the era of troponins.

The cardiac troponins are remarkably sensitive for detecting myocardial injury, more sensitive than CK. Occasionally patients demonstrate an increase in troponin when there is no evidence for coronary artery disease, so that the test may be overly sensitive. Yet troponin levels are either normal or only minimally elevated after direct current cardioversion. Cardiac troponin-T levels have been noted to be increased in patients with polymyositis, dermatomyositis, and chronic renal failure, whereas troponin I may be more specific for myocardial injury. The continuing refinement of the assays, however, is beginning to indicate that the two have fairly similar sensitivities and specificities. Newer versions of the troponin-T assays are less affected by reduced renal function. However, when troponin T is increased, one must always inquire about renal function. Patients with renal dysfunction should have serial troponins measured, where an incremental change probably indicates acute myocardial necrosis.

There is no question that the development of troponin T and troponin I as markers of acute cardiac injury has been an important advance. How their use evolves in the management of patients with AMI and other coronary syndromes will require additional study. Routine serial troponin levels are not recommended, however, and troponin-negative patients still have about a 5% risk of a complicated course. Clinical context and ancillary data (ECGs, CK, and CK-MB, etc.) are always required in making decisions about the management of acute coronary syndromes.

OTHER LABORATORY STUDIES

The white blood count (WBC) and erythrocyte sedimentation rate (ESR) are usually elevated in AMI. Presumably they reflect a non-specific inflammatory response to injury. Some hospitals employ these tests routinely in the diagnosis of MI. A relative lymphocytosis may occur in the setting of acute MI and may provide prognostic information. As a rule, the WBC varies from 12,000 to 15,000 in most patients, but it may rise as high as 15,000 to 20,000. There may be a modest shift to the left. Leukocytosis usually recedes after a few days and disappears by the end of a week. Persistence of the leukocytosis or a very high WBC count (> 20,000) suggests the development of complications such as pulmonary embolism, pneumonia, or pericarditis. Sedimentation rates usually rise after the first few days following AMI and may remain elevated for many weeks. Particularly high ESR values are noted with complications such as pulmonary embolism and pericarditis.

Increased concentrations of the acute-phase reactant C-reactive protein (CRP) in patients with unstable angina or non–ST-T-elevation MI are correlated with an increased 14-day mortality.

CHEST RADIOGRAPH

Serial study of the chest radiograph in patients with AMI is particularly helpful, especially in evaluating the temporal sequence of hemodynamic changes. One should remember that most chest films obtained in the CCU employ the portable anteroposterior technique, which tends to magnify heart size to some extent and makes the diagnosis of cardiomegaly less reliable. For patients who are not critically ill, one should ask the x-ray technician to take a 6-foot posteroanterior chest radiograph with the patient sitting upright on the edge of the bed and the film shot from behind. The degree of congestion and left heart size on the initial chest x-ray following AMI may be particularly useful for defining prognostic groups.

Transduction of fluid from the pulmonary capillaries into the interstitial space occurs when the pulmonary capillary wedge (PCW) pressure exceeds 25 mm Hg. In fact, interstitial pulmonary edema may occur at lower wedge pressures when there has been damage to the capillary membranes. Interstitial pulmonary edema manifests roentgenographically by Kerley "B" lines, which have been reported to occur with left atrial pressure as low as 14 mm Hg but usually require a PCW pressure of 18 to 25 mm Hg. Redistribution of flow to the apices, loss of the sharp marginal contour of the pulmonary vessels, development of perihilar haze, and periacinar rosette formation are other radiologic signs of pulmonary vascular congestion and elevated PCW pressure. Pulmonary venous distention is not a reliable index of acute cardiac failure, since chest films in patients with AMI are not usually of a quality sufficient to evaluate pulmonary vessels.

In roughly 40% of patients with AMI who develop pulmonary edema, there will be radiographic evidence of pulmonary congestion before rales or other clinical signs of left heart failure are present. However, in most cases, the left ventricular decompensation requires up to 12 hours to manifest itself radiographically. In the latter situation, it is possible for the patient to receive immediate, successful therapy for early decompensation only to have "roentgenographic" pulmonary edema appear after the wedge pressure has returned to normal (see McHugh et al. in the bibliography at the end of this chapter). This may lead to the overuse of potent diuretics, resulting in hypovolemia and even shock.

Additionally, there can be a "post-therapeutic"–phase lag, which refers to the time required for the chest film to normalize following the treatment of elevated wedge pressure. This phenomenon is due to the time required for edema fluid to be reabsorbed when the wedge pressure drops with treatment. This resorption of fluid may take up to 4 days, and again can lead to the wrong decision [i.e., continued use of potent diuretics (see Kostuk et al. and McHugh et al. in the bibliography)]. The physician should also be aware that chronic interstitial fibrosis can masquerade as interstitial edema.

MYOCARDIAL IMAGING

Myocardial perfusion imaging with technetium-99m sestamibi is a very sensitive means of visualizing acute myocardial infarction. When it is injected within 6 hours after the onset of chest pain, a myocardial perfusion defect will be visualized at the infarct location. This defect can be observed in both Q-wave and non-Q-wave AMI. The perfusion abnormality is diminished over time, and when the time interval between onset of pain and isotope injection is greater than 6 hours, the perfusion image may be normal. Spontaneous thrombolysis or thrombolytic therapy may also decrease the perfusion abnormality. Therefore, when used in the setting of AMI, sestamibi should be injected before the start of thrombolytic therapy; then, even though the imaging is carried out much later, the image represents regional myocardial blood flow at the time of injection. This is because sestamibi undergoes negligible redistribution. The sestamibi scan in essence depicts the area at risk in patients with AMI. Repeat sestamibi injection and imaging after thrombolysis can then determine the salvage of myocardium by successful reperfusion. The size of the sestamibi defect soon after thrombolysis correlates well with measurement of left ventricular ejection fraction at the time of discharge from the hospital.

Sestamibi scans are sometimes performed in the emergency department to assess patients with chest pain who fail to demonstrate ECG criteria for thrombolytic therapy. If a large myocardial perfusion defect is demonstrated, thrombolytic therapy may be justified. Acute myocardial ischemia can also be visualized in the emergency department with sestamibi scanning, where it may prove helpful in distinguishing non-cardiac pain from acute coronary syndromes. Sestamibi imaging of the heart in patients with presumed acute MI remains an attractive strategy, but patients should be highly selected, as it is a relatively expensive tool.

RADIONUCLIDE VENTRICULOGRAPHY

Radionuclide ventriculography (RVG) is sometimes used in patients with AMI to assess LV function, but it has been largely replaced by echocardiography. Imaging by echo is usually more readily available, is completely non-invasive, and is perhaps more effective in demonstrating segmental dysfunction, valvular abnormalities, and cardiac thrombi. Nevertheless, RVGs continue to be performed in some centers as the method of choice in evaluating post-MI left ventricular (LV) function. Both the equilibrium technique and the first-pass method can be used to obtain radioactive counts during the cardiac cycle, from which an ejection fraction can be calculated with the assistance of a computer. The normal ejection fraction is $62 \pm 12\%$. Because there is substantial day-to-day variability in the ejection fraction during the first few days following acute MI, and because the left ventricle may later recover function following a "stunned" period of several days, it is usually better to wait until the patient has more fully recovered before evaluating global systolic function with this technique. It is best used at or near the time of discharge, when information about ejection fraction may have more prognostic value. It is currently not considered a routine test but may be valuable in selected patients.

Echocardiography

The echocardiogram has emerged as the imaging technique of choice for the assessment of cardiac size and function in the setting of AMI. It is readily available, completely non-invasive, can be repeated frequently if needed, and provides exquisite information regarding LV-segmental function, LV and right ventricular (RV) size and shape, valvular structure and function, and intra-cardiac thrombi. Echocardiography is frequently employed in the emergency department to confirm or exclude the diagnosis of acute myocardial infarction. It is particularly helpful in patients with suspected ventricular septal rupture, acute onset of mitral regurgitation or RV infarct. In general, patients with acute infarction who develop increasingly severe pump dysfunction should undergo echocardiography in order to help determine the mechanism of the low-cardiac-output state. In such cases, consideration should be given to the diagnosis of pericardial tamponade, myocardial rupture, ventricular septal rupture, acute mitral regurgitation due to papillary muscle dysfunction or a flail mitral valve leaflet, RV infarct, massive pulmonary embolus, or "power failure" due to severe global LV dysfunction. Disruption of the mitral valve apparatus is best visualized by transesophageal echocardiography (TEE), as is acute ventricular septal defect. An additional benefit of echocardiography is identification of LV thrombus. Thrombi that are mobile and pedunculated are more likely to embolize and therefore require urgent anticoagulation. RV infarct is characterized by a severely dysfunctional and sometimes dilated right ventricle. Large pulmonary emboli are also characterized by a dilated, dysfunctional right ventricle. Right-sided ECG leads may be used to help distinguish these two entities (see Chapter 26). Although echocardiography is increasingly being used as an important tool to guide diagnosis and therapy in patients with acute infarction, it should not be considered a routine test to be performed daily on each and every patient. It will prove to be most valuable when used in those patients suspected of having specific mechanical or thromboembolic complications. It is important to recognize that the echocardiogram performed on day 1 of a MI may show profound cardiac depression, which may then improve substantially over several days. Early marked impairment of ventricular function may be due to myocardial stunning, which resolves over subsequent days.

PROTOCOL

1. Total CK and CK-MB isoenzyme activity should be measured on admission and 12 and 24 hours later until three samples have been obtained.

   For patients arriving late after the onset of chest pain, in whom the CK elevation might have been missed (e.g., 3 to 4 days after the index event), troponin T or troponin I should be ordered.

   Troponin T or troponin I is the marker of choice for AMI in most hospitals. These markers are usually increased by 3 hours after chest pain and may stay elevated for 11 days post-MI. They are more sensitive and specific than CK and CK-MB. Troponin T can be affected by renal insufficiency or renal failure.

2. A 12-lead ECG should be ordered on admission and daily for the first 3 days. Instructions should also be given to obtain a 12-lead ECG along with a recording of the heart rate and blood pressure during episodes of chest pain.

3. A portable chest radiograph should be ordered on admission. Additional chest films should be obtained daily in the CCU or if the patient's clinical condition alters (e.g., pulmonary edema, hypotension).

4. Radionuclide myocardial sestamibi imaging may be a useful adjunct in the diagnosis of AMI in selected patients.

5. Radionuclide ventriculography may be useful in selected patients at the time of discharge.

6. Echocardiography offers valuable information about the size, shape, and performance of the heart and allows one to visualize LV thrombi. It is now the imaging test of choice for patients with AMI. It should be performed prior to discharge to characterize cardiac function, size, and shape and to provide information regarding valvular dysfunction and intracardiac thrombi.

BIBLIOGRAPHY

Adams, J.E. III, Abendschein, D.R., and Jaffe, A.S. Biochemical markers of myocardial injury: is MB creatine kinase the choice for the 1990s? *Circulation.* 88:750–763, 1993.

Antman, E.M., Tanasijevic, M.J., Thompson, B., et al. Cardiac-specific troponin I levels to predict the risk of mortality in patients with acute coronary syndromes. *N. Engl. J. Med.* 335:1342–1349, 1996.

Aldrich, H.R., Wagner, N.B., Boswick, J., et al. Use of initial ST-segment deviation for prediction of final electrocardiographic size of acute myocardial infarcts. *Am. J. Cardiol.* 61:749–753, 1988.

Hamm, C.W., Goldmann, B.U., Heeschen, C., et al. Emergency room triage of patients with acute chest pain by means of rapid testing for cardiac troponin T or troponin I. *N. Engl. J. Med.* 337:1648–1653, 1997.

Hathaway, W.R., Peterson, E.D., Wagner, G.S., et al. Prognostic significance of the initial electrocardiogram in patients with acute myocardial infarction. *J.A.M.A.* 279: 387–391, 1998.

Hochrein, J., Sun, F., Pieper, K.S., et al. Higher T-wave amplitude associated with better prognosis in patients receiving thrombolytic therapy for acute myocardial infarction (a GUSTO-1 Substudy). *Am. J. Cardiol.* 81: 1078–1084, 1998.

Kostuk, W., Barr, J.W., Simon, A.L., and Ross, J., Jr. Correlation between the chest film and hemodynamics in acute myocardial infarction. *Circulation* 48:624–632, 1982.

Langer, A., Krucoff, M.W., Klootwijk, P., et al. Prognostic significance of ST segment shift early after resolution of ST elevation in patients with myocardial infarction treated with thrombolytic therapy: the GUSTO-I ST segment monitoring substudy. *J. Am. Coll. Cardiol.* 31: 783–789, 1998.

Lee, T.H., and Goldman, L. Serum enzyme assays in the diagnosis of acute myocardial infarction. *Ann. Intern. Med.* 105:221–223, 1986.

Lee, T.H., Weiberg, M.C., Cook, E.F., et al. Evaluation of creatine kinase and creatine kinase-MB for diagnosing myocardial infarction. *Arch. Intern. Med.* 147:115–121, 1987.

Lüscher, M.S., Thygesen, K., Ravkilde, J., and Heickendorff, L. Applicability of cardiac troponin T and I for early risk stratification in unstable coronary artery disease. *Circulation.* 96:2578–2585, 1997.

McHugh, T.J., Forrester, J.S., Adler, L., Zion, D., and Swan, H.J.C. Pulmonary vascular congestion in acute myocardial infarction: Hemodynamics and radiologic correlations. *Ann. Intern. Med.* 76:29–33, 1972.

Morrow, D.A., Rifai, N., Antman, E.M., Winer, D.L., McCabe, C.H., Cannon, C.P., and Braunwald, E. C-reactive protein is a potent predictor of mortality independently of and in combination with troponin T in acute coronary syndromes: A TIMI 11A substudy. *J. Am. Coll. Cardiol.* 31:1460–1465, 1998.

Olatidoye, A.G., Wu, A.H.B., Feng, Y-J., Waters, D. Prognostic role of troponin T versus troponin I in unstable angina pectoris for cardiac events with meta-analysis comparing published studies. *Am. J. Cardiol.* 81:1405–1410, 1998.

Phibbs, B., Marcus, F., Marriot, H.J.C., Moss, A., and Spodick, D.H. Q-wave versus non-Q-wave myocardial infarction: A meaningless distinction. *J. Am. Coll. Cardiol.* 33: 576–582, 1999.

Quinones, M.A. Echocardiography in acute myocardial infarction. *Cardiol. Clin.* 2:123–134, 1984.

Sgarbossa, E.B., Pinski, S.L., Barbagelata, A., et al. Electrocardiographic diagnosis of evolving acute myocardial infarction in the presence of left bundle-branch block. *N. Engl. J. Med.* 334:481–487, 1996.

Shah, A., Wagner, G.S., Califf, R.M., et al. Comparative prognostic significance of simultaneous versus independent resolution of ST segment depression relative to ST segment elevation during acute myocardial infarction. *J. Am. Coll. Cardiol.* 30:1478–1483, 1997.

White, R.D., Grande, P., Califf, L., Palmeri, S.T., Califf, R.M., and Wagner, G.S. Diagnostic and prognostic significance in minimally elevated creatine kinase-MB in suspected acute myocardial infarction. *Am. J. Cardiol.* 55: 1478–1484, 1985.

Yusuf, S., Collins, R., Lin, L., Sterry, H., Pearson, M., and Sleight, P. Significance of elevated MB isoenzyme with normal creatine kinase in acute myocardial infarction. *Am. J. Cardiol.* 59:245–250, 1987.

12

Modification of Myocardial Infarction Size

A variety of hemodynamic and pharmacologic interventions have been found to alter infarct size in experimental animal models of myocardial infarction (MI). A number of these interventions have been utilized in patients with acute MI (AMI) with considerable success. The best form of infarct size reduction involves re-opening (thrombolysis) the thrombosed coronary artery that led to infarction (see Chapter 13).

ALTERATION IN MYOCARDIAL OXYGEN DEMAND
Myocardial oxygen demand is a major factor in the survival of myocardial cells made critically ischemic (although still viable) during an acute infarction (see Chapter 1 and Fig. 12-1). Clearly, factors that increase myocardial oxygen consumption will adversely affect such cells, and vice versa. Animal studies have demonstrated that tachycardia and positive inotropic agents such as isoproterenol, digitalis, and glucagon have an adverse effect on infarct size in nonfailing hearts. In failing hearts, digitalis reduces infarct size, presumably by decreasing left ventricular dilatation and hence wall stress. Wall stress is one of the three major factors that determine myocardial oxygen consumption. The other two factors are heart rate and contractility (see Chapter 1). Beta-adrenergic blocking agents reduce myocardial oxygen consumption and have been reported to reduce infarct size in both animals and humans; major clinical trials of beta blockade in AMI have demonstrated reduced infarct size as well as mortality.

Intra-aortic balloon counterpulsation has been shown to reduce experimental infarct size, partly by reducing left ventricular work and hence myocardial oxygen demand and partly by increasing myocardial blood flow (see Chapter 28).

The routine use of beta-blocking agents in all patients with AMI is indicated unless patients have strong contraindications to beta blockade, e.g., asthma. Measures aimed at reducing tachycardia and left ventricular wall stress, such as treatment of hypertension, volume depletion, heart failure, anxiety, and agitation, are also clearly indicated. The use of isoproterenol under any circumstance, and of digitalis in nonfailing hearts, should be avoided.

In the absence of contraindications (history of asthma or wheezing, heart block, marked left ventricular failure), the

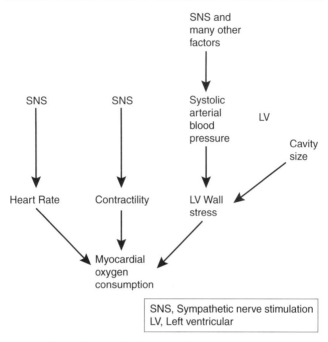

Figure 12-1.   Myocardial oxygen demand.

following classes of patients with AMI should be strongly considered for beta-blocker therapy:

1. All patients with Q-wave and non-Q-wave MI.
2. Patients with angina pectoris following Q-wave or non-Q-wave MI.
3. Patients who are hypertensive during the first 4 to 6 hours after MI. Patients who become hypertensive at a later phase of their recuperation should also be considered for beta blockade (see Chapter 22).
4. Patients who demonstrate tachycardia or near tachycardia (heart rate in excess of 80 beats per minute) and who do not have marked heart failure or hypotension.

Patients who receive beta-blocker therapy early in the course of AMI should have this therapy initiated by the intravenous route—e.g., metoprolol 5 mg IV q5min × 3. Thereafter, oral therapy can be titrated to maintain the heart rate at <55 beats per minute and the systolic blood pressure <120 mm Hg if tolerated.

IMPROVEMENT IN MYOCARDIAL BLOOD FLOW

Thrombolysis is the most effective way to reestablish myocardial blood flow to an infarcting region of myocardium (Chapter 13). Also, as noted above, counterpulsation has been shown to reduce experimental infarct size. Two mechanisms are operative here: decreased left ventricular oxygen demand and increased myocardial blood flow. Similarly, nitroglycerin reduces infarct size in animals and possibly in humans. The mechanism of nitroglycerin's beneficial effect is still contested but is probably secondary to decreased myocardial oxygen consumption. Nitroglycerin reduces left ventricular cavity size and hence wall tension by dilating large-capacitance veins and pooling blood in the periphery. Increased myocardial blood flow can also occur through collateral blood vessels because of the drug's direct vasodilating properties and because reduced left ventricular wall tension lessens systolic compression of collateral blood vessels. It is common practice to place patients with adequate arterial blood pressure (systolic arterial pressure > 100 mm Hg) on intravenous nitroglycerin for 48 to 72 hours.

Angioplasty and/or coronary artery bypass surgery (CABG) can increase myocardial blood flow. But CABG can rarely be performed rapidly enough (within hours) following acute infarction to affect infarct size. Routine counterpulsation is not advised in acute infarction.

AUGMENTATION OF ENERGY SOURCES IN ISCHEMIC MYOCARDIUM

Increased levels of glucose, insulin, and potassium made available to anoxic heart preparations improve myocardial function, presumably secondary to the increased intracellular levels of high-energy phosphates that result from this "forced feeding" of myocardial cells. The intravenous glucose-insulin-potassium regimen of Sodi-Pallares has been shown to reduce infarct size in animals. Clinical trials have produced mixed results; and therefore one cannot yet advise the routine use of this program in the treatment of MI. It seems reasonable, however, to provide such patients with a diet high in glucose and potassium (see Chapter 6).

IMPROVED DIFFUSION OF OXYGEN AND SUBSTRATES TO ISCHEMIC CELLS

Initial observations indicated that experimental and clinical infarct size could be reduced by means of intravenous hyaluronidase therapy, presumably because this agent increased diffusion through the extracellular space and hence might facilitate delivery of substrates to ischemic cells. However, randomized trials in patients with AMI did not support the concept that hyaluronidase administration reduced infarct size in humans, and the use of this agent has ceased.

Supplemental inspiratory oxygen has been shown to decrease infarct size in animals and humans, presumably by increasing the diffusion of oxygen into ischemic areas of myocardium. These results support the current practice of administering supplemental inspiratory oxygen to patients with acute infarction (see Chapter 10).

BIBLIOGRAPHY

Bussmann, W.D., Passek, D., Seidel, W., and Kaltenback, M. Reduction of CK and CK-MB indexes of infarct size by intravenous nitroglycerin. *Circulation* 63:615–622, 1981.

Bussmann, W.D., Seher, W., and Gruengras, M. Reduction of creatine kinase and creatine kinase-MB indexes of infarct size by intravenous verapamil. *Am. J. Cardiol.* 54:1224–1230, 1984.

Diaz, R., Paolasso, E.A., Piegas, L.S., Tajer, C.D., Moreno, M.G., Corvalan, R., et al. Metabolic modulation of acute myocardial infarction—The ECLA glucose-insulin-potassium pilot trial. *Circulation* 98:2227–2234, 1998.

Epstein, S.E., Kent, K.M., Goldstein, R.E., Boyer, J.S., and Redwood, D.R. Reduction of ischemic injury by nitroglycerin during acute myocardial infarction. *N. Engl. J. Med.* 292:29–35, 1975.

Maroko, P.R., and Braunwald, E. Modification of myocardial infarction size after coronary occlusion. *Ann. Intern. Med.* 79:720–733, 1973.

Ordoubadi-Fath, F., and Beatt, K.J. Glucose-insulin-potassium therapy for treatment of acute myocardial infarction—An overview of randomized placebo-controlled trials. *Circulation* 96:1152–1156, 1997.

Roberts, R., et al. Effect of propranolol on myocardial infarct size in randomized blinded multicenter trial. *N. Engl. J. Med.* 311:218–225, 1984.

Rogers, W.J., Segall, P.H., McDaniel, H.G., Mantle, J.A., Russell, R.O., and Rackley, C.E. Prospective randomized trial of glucose-insulin-potassium in acute myocardial infarction: Effects of myocardial hemodynamics, substrates and rhythm. *Am. J. Cardiol.* 48:801–809, 1979.

Ryan, T.J., Anderson, J.L., Antman, E.M., Braniff, B.A., Brooks, N.H., Califf, R.M., et al. ACC/AHA Guidelines for the management of patients with acute myocardial infarction. *J. Am. Coll. Cardiol.* 28:1328–1428, 1996.

Savage, R.M., Guth, B., White, F.C., Hagan, A.D., and Bloor, C.M. Correlation of regional myocardial blood flow and function with myocardial infarct size during acute myocardial ischemia and the conscious pig. *Circulation* 64: 699–707, 1981.

The International Collaborative Study Group. Acute myocardial infarct size reduction by timolol administration. *Am. J. Cardiol.* 57:28F–33F, 1986.

Wetstein, L., Simson, M.B., Feldman, P.D., and Harken, A.H. Pharmacologic modification of myocardial ischemia. *Circulation* 66:548–554, 1982.

13

Coronary Reperfusion—
Pharmacologic
and Mechanical

Intravenous thrombolytic trials have now enrolled more than 250,000 cumulative patients and the results indicate a reduction in 30-day mortality from 15% to 7.5%. The benefit persists for years. The use of thrombolytic therapy is predicated on the now secure concept that acute transmural myocardial infarction (AMI) with ST-T–segment elevation is associated with the development of fresh thrombus, often superimposed on a ruptured plaque of an epicardial coronary artery. Coronary atherosclerotic disease is the underlying substrate in nearly all patients with AMI. Approximately 1 million patients come to the hospital each year in the United States with AMI. About 200,000 patients receive "reperfusion therapy" in the United States each year. The time to treatment is a pivotal parameter in successful reperfusion. Patients treated in the first 4 hours have the greatest benefit, while there is little or no benefit for patients treated at 12 hours or beyond.

There are currently three commonly used protocols for pharmacologic reperfusion.

PROTOCOL
1. Patients who fulfill the following criteria are candidates for coronary thrombolysis.
   a. Chest pain at rest compatible with acute myocardial ischemia for *less than 4 to 6 hours* (exact time limits are still debated; many cardiologists treat up to 12 hours after the onset of pain).
      (1) Unrelieved by a nitrate preparation
      (2) Without obvious non-cardiac explanation
   b. Electrocardiogram that reveals one of the following findings:
      (1) New or presumably new ST-segment elevation ≥ 0.1 mV in two or more contiguous leads
      (2) Left bundle-branch block
2. Patients are excluded from entrance into either study for the following reasons:
   a. Presence of active bleeding

   b. History of recent (within 2 months) stroke, intracranial or intraspinal surgery
   c. Known intracranial neoplasm or symptoms compatible with space occupying central nervous system (CNS) lesion
   d. Recent (within 10 days) major surgery or gastrointestinal bleeding
   e. Recent trauma, including prolonged cardiopulmonary resuscitation
   f. Severe uncontrolled arterial hypertension (systolic BP > 180 mm Hg)
   g. Known severe hemostatic defects, known severe liver or renal disease
   h. Prior use of streptokinase, which eliminates its re-use
3. Accelerated alteplase tissue plasminogen activator (t-PA) over 90 minutes administered with intravenous heparin.
   a. Bolus dose of 15 mg t-PA followed by an infusion of 0.75 mg/kg over 30 minutes (not to exceed 50 mg) and an infusion of 0.5 mg/kg (up to 35 mg) over the next 60 minutes (<100 mg over 90 minutes).
   b. IV heparin bolus of 5000 units and an initial infusion of 1000 U/h for patients weighing >67 kg.
   c. Heparin is titrated to an activated partial thromboplastin time (a PTT) of 50 to 75 seconds; PTT is measured at 6, 12, and 24 hours as well as 6 hours after change of dose. For patients ≤ 67 kg, heparin is given as a weight-adjusted 80 U/kg bolus and 18 U/kg per hour infusion. The heparin is given before or as soon as possible after the thrombolytic therapy and is continued for 48 to 72 hours.
4. Reteplase in two bolus doses of 10 units given 30 minutes apart. Heparin is given as with t-PA.
5. Streptokinase 1.5 million units over 60 minutes. No heparin is given. Streptokinase can be given only once to a patient and is more likely to cause hypotension.

In each case, non-enteric-coated aspirin 324 mg is also given unless there is a contraindication. The daily maintenance dose of 160 to 324 mg aspirin is then given daily. Intravenous and PO beta-adrenergic blockers are also given, as described in Chapter 15. t-PA and reteplase are much more expensive than streptokinase ($2200 versus $300). The dosage regimen of front-loaded t-PA is somewhat cumbersome, whereas reteplase is quite simple to give. Tenecteplase (TNK) t-PA is a genetically engineered third-generation variant of t-PA that can be given as a single weight-adjusted bolus. Both TNK and lanoteplase (NPA) are more convenient than t-PA and can be given by a single rapid injection. As of this time, they do not have FDA approval. However, it seems likely that more convenient single-dose rapid-injection TNK or NPA thrombolytic therapy will emerge as the preferred treatment.

Only about 50% to 60% of patients given thrombolytic therapy demonstrate TIMI-3 (excellent) flow at 90 minutes. Paradoxically, thrombolytic therapy is prothrombotic because free thrombin is exposed following lysis of fibrin. Thrombin strongly promotes platelet aggregation, which is resistant to thrombolytic therapy. This concept has spurred the idea of combining platelet glycoprotein (GP) *IIb*/*IIIa* platelet inhibitors with lower-dose thrombolytic therapy for the treatment of AMI, a strategy currently being tested in phase III clinical trials.

Major bleeding complications occur in about 5% of patients treated for AMI. About 0.70% of patients develop intracranial hemorrhage (ICH) during hospitalization for AMI, and 50% to 60% of those die during hospitalization. Factors predisposing to ICH include older age, female sex, a wide pulse pressure on presentation to the emergency department, black ethnicity, systolic blood pressure > 140 mm Hg, diastolic blood pressure >100 mm Hg, history of previous stroke, and low body weight. It is unknown whether reducing blood pressure prior to thrombolytic therapy is helpful in reducing ICH. The protocol for suspected ICH is as follows:

PROTOCOL

1. Discontinue thrombolytic therapy immediately.
2. Discontinue heparin and aspirin.
3. Begin volume expansion.
4. Urgent computed tomography (CT) scan of the head.
5. If the CT scan of the head indicates ICH:
   a. Give protamine if the patient has received heparin in the previous 4 hours; give 1 mg protamine for every 100 units of heparin infused during the previous 4 hours.
   b. Infuse 10 units of cryoprecipitate to replenish fibrinogen and factor VIII levels.

c.   Check fibrinogen level before and after 10 units of cryoprecipitate; target fibrinogen > 1.0 g/L.
d.   Give 2 units of fresh frozen plasma to replenish alpha$_2$-antitrypsin levels.

Cryoprecipitate may have to be re-infused if the fibrinogen level is < 1 g/L. If neurologic deterioration continues, consider giving 10 units of platelets. A CT scan of the head may be repeated when intra-vascular coagulation has been stabilized. The case should be reviewed with a neurologist and neuroradiologist. Persistent bleeding may require the use of epsilon amino-caproic acid (Amicar) 0.1 g/kg IV over 30 to 60 minutes followed by 0.5 to 1.0 g/h by infusion.

RESCUE ANGIOPLASTY
When thrombolytic therapy fails, there is need to consider "rescue angioplasty." Failure of thrombolysis is difficult to define but usually includes:

1.   Deteriorating clinical condition despite thrombolytic therapy.
2.   Chest discomfort that does not resolve or returns after resolving.
3.   Less than a 25% to 50% reduction in the sum of all leads with ST elevation or in the single worst lead. The electrocardiogram (ECG) should be repeated at 40 and 120 minutes after thrombolysis to look for evidence of reperfusion.

Rescue angioplasty refers to the use of percutaneous transluminal angioplasty (PTCA)/stenting of the culprit artery in patients in whom reperfusion has not occurred after thrombolysis. On the basis of observational data, most clinicians favor a policy of early percutaneous coronary intervention (PCI) in patients with failure to reperfuse.

REPERFUSION (PRIMARY MECHANICAL ANGIOPLASTY/STENTING)
Percutaneous coronary intervention (PCI) was first used for the treatment of AMI in the early 1980s and was popularized in the 1990s, after clinical trials demonstrated its superiority over thrombolytic therapy. There is considerable advantage of primary PCI over thrombolytic therapy in avoidance of hemorrhagic stroke. Previously, the problem of coronary restenosis explained lack of long-term efficacy of primary PTCA, but the addition of stenting has remarkably changed this, along with the use of GP IIb/IIIa antagonists

in the catheterization laboratory. The door-to-balloon time is critical, and to achieve a time of ≤ 60 minutes requires particular streamlining and readiness that is not typically encountered. A door-to-balloon time > 90 minutes is probably too long, and thrombolytic therapy should be considered rather than primary PCI in such conditions. Use of GP IIb/IIIa antagonists and stenting of culprit vessels has become commonplace. When a GP IIb/IIIa antagonist is given in the lab, the heparin infusion should be reduced to 50 U/g and the activating clotting time (ACT) should be titrated to approximately 225 seconds.

Patients with prior AMI who have had coronary artery bypass grafts (CABG) with saphenous vein graft occlusion are poor responders to thrombolytic therapy. PCI is the preferred strategy if it is available.

Although earlier studies indicated no advantage or even a disadvantage for the strategy of thrombolysis followed by early PCI, the situation has now changed. This is because of the use of new agents such as abciximab (a GP IIb/IIIa antagonist), better stents, and clopidogrel, which allow the culprit artery to be opened widely with excellent TIMI-3 flow and a low subsequent incidence of MI, unstable angina, restenosis, or death. More changes in how thrombolytic therapy and PCI are used can be expected as new trials are completed.

BIBLIOGRAPHY

Antoniucci, D., Santoro, G.M., Bolognese, L., et al. A clinical trial comparing primary stenting of the infarct-related artery with optimal primary angioplasty for acute myocardial infarction. FRESCO trial. *J. Am. Coll. Cardiol.* 31: 1234–1239, 1998.

Brener, S.J., Barr, L.A., Burchena, J.E.B., et al. Randomized, placebo-controlled trial of platelet glycoprotein IIb/IIIa blockade with primary angioplasty for acute myocardial infarction: The RAPPORT investigators. *Circulation* 98: 734–741, 1998.

Davies, C.H., and Ormerod, O.J.M. Failed coronary thrombolysis. *Lancet* 351: 1191–1196, 1998.

Doorey, A.J., Michelson, E.L., and Topol, E.J. Thrombolytic therapy of myocardial infarction. *J.A.M.A.* 268:3108–3114, 1992.

Every, N.R., Parsons, L.S., Hlatky, M., et al. A comparison of thrombolytic therapy with primary coronary angioplasty for acute myocardial infarction: MITI Investigators *N. Engl. J. Med.* 335(17): 1253–1318, 1996.

The GUSTO IIb investigators. A clinical trial comparing primary coronary angioplasty with tissue plasminogen activator for acute myocardial infarction. *N. Engl. J. Med.* 336:1621–1628, 1997.

The GUSTO III investigators. A comparison of reteplase with alteplase for acute myocardial infarction. *N. Engl. J. Med.* 337(16): 1117–1161, 1997.

Ross, A.M., Conor, F.L., and Lundergan, C.F. Rescue angioplasty after failed thrombolysis—Technical and clinical outcomes in a large thrombolysis trial: The GUSTO-1 angiographic investigators. *J. Am. Coll. Cardiol.* 31: 1511–1517, 1998.

Suryapranata, H., Hof, A.W.J.V., Hoorntje, J.C.A., de Boer, M., and Zijlstra, F. Randomized comparison of coronary stenting with balloon angioplasty in selected patients with acute myocardial infarction. *Circulation* 97: 2502–2505, 1998.

Weaver, W.D., Simes, J., Betriu, A., et al. Comparison of primary coronary angioplasty and intravenous thrombolytic therapy for acute myocardial infarction. *J.A.M.A.* 278: 2093–2098.

White, H.D., and Van de Werf, F.J.J. Thrombolysis for acute myocardial infarction. *Circulation* 97: 1632–1646, 1998.

14

Anticoagulants in Acute Myocardial Infarction

All patients with acute coronary syndromes—including unstable angina, non-S-T–wave elevation myocardial infarction (MI), and ST-wave elevation MI—should be considered for treatment with anticoagulation unless contraindicated (e.g., the presence of active bleeding or very recent surgery). Patients should be given aspirin 324 mg PO as soon as the diagnosis is suspected and daily thereafter. This should be continued indefinitely, although a lower dose of 80 mg per day may be adequate for long-term therapy. Enteric-coated aspirin should be avoided in patients with acute MI (AMI), as it takes longer to be absorbed. Chewable aspirin is preferred as initial treatment, as absorption may be faster. For patients who cannot take aspirin, clopidogrel 75 mg per day after a 300-mg loading dose may suffice. In brief, aspirin plays a fundamental role in the treatment of both unstable angina and acute MI, although it is a relatively weak anti-platelet agent.

If streptokinase is used, heparin does not appear to be routinely needed. However, heparin is given to patients who are managed with thrombolytic therapy or primary percutaneous coronary intervention. Heparin is given before or as soon as possible after the thrombolytic therapy:

INTRAVENOUS HEPARIN
5000 units IV bolus followed by a maintenance infusion of 1000 U/h for patients weighing > 67 kg (for patients weighing ≤ 67 kg, give 80 U/kg bolus followed by 18 U/kg/h maintenance infusion).

Check aPTT at 6, 12, and 24 hours and at 6 hours after any change of dose.

Target aPTT is 50 to 75 seconds.

Heparin should be continued for 48 to 72 hours.

Warfarin is best avoided, especially if invasive procedures are anticipated.

PLATELET GLYCOPROTEIN IIB/IIIA ANTAGONISTS
There is a growing awareness that the platelet glycoprotein (GP) II_b/III_a antagonists may play an important role in the management of patients with acute coronary syndromes, particularly those at high risk with persistent chest discomfort, non-ST-T–wave elevation MI, or unstable angina with

positive serum troponin levels. The short-acting agents tirofiban (Aggrastat) and eptifibatide (Integrilin) are preferred in this setting over the much longer-acting aciximab (ReoPro). They are given in conjunction with aspirin and heparin. These agents are sensitive to renal function, and their dose must be reduced in cases of renal insufficiency. They can be associated with severe thrombocytopenia, which is associated with both bleeding and ischemic events.

Eptifibatide (Integrilin) is given as a 180 µg/kg bolus followed by an infusion of 2 µg/kg/min for 72 hours. A smaller dose of 135 µg/kg bolus followed by an infusion of 0.5 µg/kg/min is used when the serum creatinine is > 4 mg/dl.

Tirofiban (Aggrastat) is given as a 0.4 µg/kg/min infusion for 30 minutes, followed by an infusion of 0.1 µg/kg/min for 48 hours.

The GP II_b/III_a antagonists must be used with great caution, if used at all, in patients with renal insufficiency. They should be avoided in patients with baseline platelet counts of less than 100,000.

There is a growing belief that the GP II_b/III_a antagonists will emerge as part of the routine management of most patients with acute MI. This hypothesis will be tested in an upcoming large clinical trial. In GUSTO IV, patients with acute MI will be randomized to half-dose of reteplase (5 and 5 units) plus an abciximab bolus and a 12-hour infusion of abciximab versus a standard treatment regimen of reteplase (10 and 10 units). Intravenous heparin will be given to both groups. The primary endpoint is 30-day mortality. Until the results of the study are known, II_b/III_a antagonists are not routinely used to treat acute ST-T–elevation MI.

LOW-MOLECULAR-WEIGHT HEPARINS

Low-molecular-weight heparins (LMWHs) are a new class of anticoagulants derived from unfractionated heparin, over which they have a number of advantages. LMWHs inhibit factor Xa, a more efficient mechanism for preventing the production of large quantities of thrombin. They have decreased sensitivity to platelet factor 4, better bioavailability, a more consistent pattern of clearance, and can be administered easily via the subcutaneous route without the need for monitoring aPTT. They also may be associated with lower rates of thrombocytopenia (heparin-induced thrombocytopenia syndrome, or HITS). The LMWHs may replace unfractionated heparin for the treatment of unstable angina and acute MI. The aPTT with LMWHs may be lower than with unfractionated heparin, but the anti-Xa to anti-II_a ratio is higher. However, the anticoagulant effects of the LMWHs cannot be quickly reversed. There has been some reluctance to use LMWH in patients destined to go to the cath lab for percutaneous coronary procedures, where unfractionated heparin is still the standard, and it can be carefully monitored. Weight-adjusted LMWH enoxaparin (Lovenox)(0.75 mg/kg by IV bolus) can be combined with abciximab in the cath lab, but experience is limited. By far most of the experience with LMWHs is outside of the setting of the cath lab. Enoxaparin is usually given as 1 mg/kg subcutaneously b.i.d. from 48 hours to a maximum of 8 days.

Other LMWHs are also being studied as possible replacements for unfractionated heparin. Daltaparin (Fragmin) is given as 120 µg/kg subcutaneously b.i.d; when given for 45 days to patients with unstable angina, it may reduce the incidence of death or AMI. It seems logical that by giving effective anti-thrombin therapy during both the acute and the chronic phases of the acute coronary syndrome additional benefit may be provided. However, the LMWHs are expensive, and more experience is needed with them in the cath lab. As experience accumulates, many believe that LMWHs will replace unfractionated heparin as the standard anti-thrombin therapy.

THROMBIN INHIBITORS

Heparin-induced thrombocytopenia syndrome (HITS) is a serious problem in the coronary care unit (CCU). Patients exposed to heparin who develop a decrease in platelet count of >50% must have heparin stopped completely. Without treatment, thromboembolic complications in HITS are fatal in 20% to 30% of patients, and about 20% require limb amputation. HITS occurs in about 1% to 2% of patients receiving heparin for 4 or more days. Lepirudin (Refludan) is a recombinant DNA biosynthetic hirudin, a direct inhibitor of thrombin. It is indicated for anti-coagulation of patients with HITS and associated thromboembolic disease in order to prevent further thromboembolic complications. Careful judgment must be used in making decisions about its use, and strict monitoring of the aPTT is necessary. The drug is excreted by the kidneys, and adjustment of the infusion rate is necessary in patients with renal impairment. Serious bleeding can occur, and there is no specific antidote.

Lepirudin

Be aware of renal and hepatic function.

Avoid this drug in patients at risk for serious bleeding, such as those with recent puncture of large vessel or organ biopsy, recent cerebrovascular accident or surgery, recent major bleeding, bacterial endocarditis, or recent use of thrombolytic or streptokinase therapy, and so on.

Do not start lepirudin in patients with baseline aPTT ratio of 2.5 or more.

The first aPTT should be done 4 hours after start of lepirudin infusion.

Follow-up aPTT determination should be done at least once daily as long as treatment with lepirudin is ongoing, and more often in patients with impaired kidney and liver function.

Target aPTT should be 1.5 to 2.5 control.

Bolus and infusion rate must be reduced when serum creatinine is > 1.5 mg/dl.

Initial usual IV bolus is 0.4 mg/kg body weight over 15 to 20 seconds, followed by a continuous infusion of 0.15 mg/kg body weight per hour.

Lepirudin is usually given for 2 to 10 days and dose is adjusted for aPTT.

PROTOCOL

1. Aspirin 324 mg/day indefinitely. Aspirin should be chewed for better absorption. Low-dose aspirin may be acceptable for longer-term chronic use.

2. Unfractionated heparin: 5000 units IV bolus followed by a maintenance infusion of 1000 U/h for patients weighing > 67 kg; for patients ≤ 67 kg, give 80 U/kg bolus followed by 18 U/kg/h maintenance infusion; target aPTT 50 to 75 s.

3. IIb/IIIa inhibitors.

   Eptifbatide (Integrilin): 180 μg/kg bolus followed by 2 μg/kg/min infusion for 72 hours. For renal impairment, reduce dose to 135 μg/kg bolus and 0.5 μ/kg/min infusion; infusion is for 48 to 72 hours.

   Tirofiban (Aggrastat): 0.4 μg/kg/min infusion for 30 minutes, followed by an infusion of 0.1 μg/kg/min for 48 hours.

4. Low-molecular-weight heparin.

   Enoxaparin (Lovenox) 1 mg/kg subcutaneously b.i.d. from 48 hours to 8 days; may be used as an alternative to unfractionated heparin.

5. Anti-thrombins.
    Lipirudin (Refludan) for HITS is usually given as an IV
    bolus 0.4 mg/kg over 12 to 20 seconds, followed by a con-
    tinuous infusion of 0.15 mg/kg/h for 2 to 10 days; dose
    adjusted for a PTT of 1.5 to 2.5 control and for renal and
    hepatic function.

BIBLIOGRAPHY

Brieger, D.B, Mak, K.H., Kotte-Marchant, K., and Topol, E.J.
    Heparin-induced thrombocytopenia. *J. Am. Coll. Card.* 31:
    1449–1459, 1998.

Cohen, M., Demers, C., Gurfinkel, E.P., et al. A comparison
    of low-molecular-weight heparin with unfractionated hep-
    arin for unstable coronary artery disease. *N. Engl. J. Med.*
    337:447–452, 1997.

Greinacher, A., Völpel, H., Janssens, U., et al. Recombinant
    hirudin (Lepirudin) provides safe and effective anticoagu-
    lation in patients with heparin-induced thrombocytope-
    nia. *Circulation* 99: 73–80, 1999.

Hirsch, J., and Fuster, V. Guide to anticoagulant therapy
    part 1: Heparin. *Circulation* 89: 1449–1468, 1994.

Hirsh, J. Heparin. *N. Engl. J. Med.* 324: 1565–1574, 1991.

Hirsh, J. Low-molecular-weight heparin. *Circulation* 98:
    1575–1582, 1998.

PRISM-PLUS Study Investigators. Inhibition of the platelet
    glycoprotein IIB/IIIa receptor with tirofiban in unstable
    angina and non-q-wave myocardial infarction. *N. Engl. J.
    Med.* 338 : 1488–1542, 1998.

PURSUIT Trial Investigators. Inhibition of platelet glyco-
    protein IIb/IIIa with eptifibatide in patients with acute
    coronary syndromes. *N. Engl. J. Med.* 339 : 436–444, 1998.

Théroux, P., Waters, D., Lam, J., Juneau, M., and McCans,
    J. Reactivation of unstable angina after the discontinua-
    tion of heparin. *N. Engl. J. Med.* 327 : 141–145, 1992.

Weitz, J.E. Low-molecular-weight heparins. *N. Engl. J.
    Med.* 337: 688–698, 1997.

15

Beta-Blocker Therapy Following Acute Myocardial Infarction

Large-scale epidemiologic trials of beta blockade in patients with recent myocardial infarction (MI) have demonstrated that these agents confer striking benefit. Well-designed double-blind trials of practolol, timolol, metoprolol, propranolol, and atenolol have all shown decreased mortality in patients receiving beta blockers as compared with control subjects. Moreover, in a number of these trials, the rate of reinfarction, the number of individuals dying suddenly, the incidence of ventricular arrhythmias, infarction size, and clinical evidence of heart failure were significantly reduced by beta-blocker therapy. These data are consistent with the previously demonstrated anti-ischemic and antiarrhythmic actions of beta blockers. Although these trials have conclusively shown that beta-blocker therapy is beneficial in patients with recent MI, a number of questions still remain: (a) Should all postinfarction patients receive these agents, or are certain groups of patients likely to obtain benefit while others are not? (b) How soon after MI should these agents be started? (c) When, if ever, can these agents be discontinued because they no longer confer benefit? The answers to these questions are currently not available, but reasonable suggestions can be made.

1. Which post-MI patients should receive beta blockers? Certain categories of infarction patients benefit more than others. Thus, individuals with mild to moderate heart failure and persistent ventricular ectopy seem to benefit more from beta blocker therapy than do individuals whose infarctions are totally uncomplicated. Patients with non-ST-T–wave elevation infarction/ unstable angina and those with positive exercise tests following infarction can also be expected to gain more marked benefit from beta-blocker therapy than individuals with uncomplicated, ST-T–wave elevation infarctions whose post-infarction exercise tests are negative for MI. As discussed in Chapters 18, 19, and 22, patients with non-Q-wave infarctions, unstable angina, or positive post-infarction exercise tests often undergo coronary arteriography to define the severity of atheroscle-

rotic lesions in order to plan invasive mechanical therapy [percutaneous transluminal angioplasty (PTCA), coronary bypass]. Beta-blocker therapy has also been shown to be of benefit when administered to patients who are receiving thrombolytic therapy.

2. How soon after MI should beta-blocker therapy be started? The Göteborg metoprolol trial and the TIMI-2 trial both demonstrated benefit from metoprolol when it was administered during the first 24 hours after the onset of MI. However, the other beta-blocker trials administered these agents days to weeks following MI and were still able to demonstrate benefit.

3. Once initiated, when, if ever, should these agents be discontinued? Although no trials have specifically asked this question, most of the epidemiologic trials have demonstrated benefit for at least 12 to 18 months and possibly longer. Beta-blocker side effects can be unpleasant, and physicians must balance expected benefit from continued therapy against the adverse reactions, such as fatigue, depression, impotence in men, and decreased mental acuity.

PROTOCOL

1. All post-infarction patients are candidates for long-term beta-blocker therapy, including individuals who are receiving thrombolytic therapy. Certain groups of patients can be expected to benefit more than others. Those classes of patients who benefit the most are as follows:

   a. Patients with infarction complicated by mild to moderate heart failure and persistent ventricular arrhythmias.

   b. Patients who have a post-infarction exercise test that is positive for myocardial ischemia.

   c. Patients with non-ST-T–wave elevation infarction/unstable angina. Many of these patients will proceed to cardiac catheterization, PTCA, and coronary bypass surgery.

   d. Some authorities do not administer beta blockers to patients with totally uncomplicated MIs.

2. Beta-blocker therapy can be administered immediately or on day 5 to 7 post-infarction.

   a. Recommended oral dosages of beta blockers are as follows:

      (1) Timolol 10 mg b.i.d.

      (2) Metoprolol 100 mg b.i.d.(widely used)

(3) Propranolol 180 to 240 mg in divided doses b.i.d. or t.i.d.

(4) Atenolol 50 to 100 mg/day

One usually attempts to reduce the heart rate to less than 75 when possible.

b. Recommended intravenous dosage is as follows:

(1) Metoprolol is initiated as 15 mg IV over 10 to 15 minutes (5 mg q5min) followed by 100 mg PO b.i.d.

The dose will vary widely from patient to patient.

(2) Propranolol is initiated as 5 to 8 mg IV over 10 to 15 minutes, followed by 180 to 240 mg PO in divided doses, b.i.d. or t.i.d. (rarely used).

(3) Atenolol is initiated as 5 mg IV over 10 minutes, followed by a second 5-mg IV dose 20 minutes later; oral atenolol is then given at 50 mg every day.

3. Beta-blocker therapy is continued for at least 12 to 18 months. Many cardiologists continue therapy indefinitely in the absence of adverse effects.

4. Beta-blocker therapy is contraindicated in infarction patients with severe heart failure (pulmonary edema), hypotension or cardiogenic shock, second- or third-degree A-V block, marked sinus bradycardia (heart rate < 50/min) and a history of bronchial asthma or bronchospastic chronic obstructive pulmonary disease.

BIBLIOGRAPHY

Beta Blocker Heart Attack Research Group. A randomized trial of propranolol in patients with acute myocardial infarction: I. Mortality results. *J.A.M.A.* 247:1707–1714, 1982.

Ellis, S.G., Muller, D.W., and Topol, E.J. Possible survival benefit from concomitant beta- but not calcium-antagonist therapy during reperfusion for acute myocardial infarction. *Am. J. Cardiol.* 66:125–128, 1990.

First International Study of Infarct Survival Collaboration Group. Randomized trial of intravenous atenolol among 16,027 cases of suspected acute myocardial infarction: ISIS-I. *Lancet* 2:57–66, 1986.

Frishman, W.H., Furberg, C.D., and Friedewald, W.T. Beta adrenergic blockade for survivors of acute myocardial infarction. *N. Engl. J. Med.* 310:830–837, 1984.

Gottlieb, S.S., McCarter, R.J., Vogel, R.A. Effect of beta blockade on mortality among high-risk and low-risk patients after myocardial infarction. *N. Engl. J. Med.* 339:489–497, 1998.

Hjalmarson, Å. The Göteborg metoprolol trial in acute myocardial infarction. *Am. J. Cardiol.* (Suppl. 6/25/84) 53: ID–50D, 1984.

Hjalmarson, Å., Olsson, G. Myocardial infarction: Effects of beta blockade. *Circulation* (Suppl. VI) 84:VI-101–VI-107, 1991.

Krumholtz, H.M., Radford, M.J., Wang, Y., Chen, J., Heiat, A., and Marciniak, T.A. National use and effectiveness of beta blockers for the treatment of elderly patients after acute myocardial infarction—National Cooperative Cardiovascular Project. *JAMA,* 280:623–629, 1998.

Lau, J., Antman, E.M., Jimenez-Silva, J., et al. Cumulative meta-analysis of therapeutic trials for myocardial infarction. *N. Engl. J. Med.* 327:248–254, 1992.

Norwegian Multicenter Study Group. Timolol-induced reduction in mortality and reinfarction in patients surviving acute myocardial infarction. *N. Engl. J. Med.* 304: 801–807, 1981.

Pedersen, T. R., and Norwegian Multicenter Study Group. Six year followup of the Norwegian multicenter study on timolol after acute myocardial infarction. *N. Engl. J. Med.* 313:1055–1058, 1985.

The MIAMI Trial Research Group. Metoprolol in acute myocardial infarction: Patient population. *Am. J. Cardiol.* 56:1G–57G, 1985.

The TIMI Study Group. Comparison of invasive and conservative strategies after treatment with intravenous tissue plasminogen activator in acute myocardial infarction: Results of the thrombolysis in myocardial infarction (TIMI) phase II trial. *N. Engl. J. Med.* 320:618–627, 1989.

Yusuf, S., Peto, R., Lewis, J., Collins, R., and Sleight, P. Beta blockade during and after myocardial infarction: An overview of the randomized trials. *Prog. Cardiovasc. Dis.* 27:335–371, 1985.

16

Calcium Channel Blockers in Acute Myocardial Infarction

Calcium channel blockers (CCBs) have a number of pharmacologic properties that should theoretically confer benefit to patients with acute myocardial infarction (AMI), such as reduction of blood pressure (all CCBs), heart rate (diltiazem, verapamil), and myocardial contractility (all CCBs), together with coronary vasodilation (all CCBs). Indeed, in experimental animal models of AMI, CCBs have been shown to reduce infarct size, increase coronary collateral blood flow, stabilize ischemic myocardial cells, and decrease ventricular premature contractions. On the basis of these potentially beneficial properties and promising experimental results, CCBs were employed in a number of clinical trials involving patients with AMI. The results have generally been disappointing.

Nifedipine and its analogs (the dihydropyridines) failed to demonstrate any benefit; indeed, harm occurred in some studies. Verapamil and diltiazem conferred benefit in post-MI patients who were without clinical evidence of heart failure. In patients with heart failure following MI, no benefit was observed, and even possible harm occurred with diltiazem. Diltiazem has been shown, however, to reduce unstable angina and reinfarction in patients with recent non-ST–wave elevation MI. All CCBs have been shown to be beneficial when added to beta blockers for patients with unstable angina following AMI. In these studies, the CCBs were started 3 to 4 days or more following the onset of the acute myocardial infarct.

PROTOCOL

1. In general, beta blockers are preferred to CCBs in AMI.
2. CCBs can be of benefit when added to beta-blocker therapy in patients with unstable angina with or without recent MI.
3. With respect to chronic drug therapy following AMI:
   a. In patients with ST-T–wave elevation infarction without heart failure or significant left ventricular dysfunction (LVEF > 40%), beta blockers are preferred.
   b. In patients with ST-T–wave elevation infarction with heart failure or significant left ventricular dys-

function (LVEF < 40%), CCBs should be avoided.
Beta blockers can often be safely administered.

c. In patients with non-ST-T–wave elevation infarction
or unstable angina without heart failure or significant left ventricular dysfunction (LVEF > 40%), diltiazem, verapamil, or beta blockers can be employed.

d. In patients with non-Q-wave infarction or unstable
angina with heart failure or significant left ventricular dysfunction (LVEF < 40%), CCBs should be
avoided.

BIBLIOGRAPHY

Danish Study Group on Verapamil in Myocardial Infarction.
Effect of verapamil on mortality and major events after
acute myocardial infarction (The Danish verapamil infarction trial II—DAVIT II). *Am. J. Cardiol.* 66:779–784,
1990.

Danish Study Group on Verapamil in Myocardial Infarction.
Secondary prevention with verapamil after myocardial
infarction. *Am. J. Cardiol.* 66:331–401, 1990.

Danish Study Group on Verapamil in Myocardial Infarction.
Verapamil in acute myocardial infarction. *Eur. Heart J.*
5:516–528, 1984.

Furberg, C.D., Psaty, B.M., and Meyer, J.V. Nifedipine:
Dose-related increase in mortality in patients with coronary heart disease. *Circulation* 92:1326–1331, 1995.

Gibson, R.S. Current status of calcium channel-blocking
drugs after Q wave and non-Q wave myocardial infarction.
Circulation 80 (suppl. IV):107–119, 1989.

Held, P.H., Yusuf, S., and Furberg, C.D. Calcium-channel
blockers in acute myocardial infarction and unstable
angina: An overview. *Br. Med. J.* 299:1187–1192, 1989.

Ishikawa, K., Nakai, S., Takenaka, T., Kanamasa, K.,
Hama, J., Ogawa, I., et al. Short-acting nifedipine and diltiazem do not reduce the incidence of cardiac events in
patients with healed myocardial infarction. *Circulation*
95:2368–2373, 1997.

Moss, A.J. Secondary prevention with calcium channel-
blocking drugs in patients after myocardial infarction: A
critical review. *Circulation* 75 (suppl V):V148–V153, 1987.

Roberts, R. Review of calcium antagonist trials in acute
myocardial infarction. *Clin. Cardiol.* 12:41–47, 1989.

Skolnick, A.E., and Frishman, W.H. Calcium channel blockers in myocardial infarction. *Arch. Intern. Med.* 146:
1669–1677, 1989.

The Israeli SPRINT Study Group. Secondary prevention reinfarction Israeli nifedipine trial (SPRINT): A randomized intervention trial of nifedipine in patients with acute myocardial infarction. *Eur. Heart J.* 9:354–364, 1988.

The Multicenter Diltiazem Postinfarction Trial Research Group. The effect of diltiazem on mortality and reinfarction after myocardial infarction. *N. Engl. J. Med.* 319: 385–392, 1988.

Theroux, P., Gregoire, J., Chin, C., Pelletier, G., deGuise, P., and Juneau, M. Intravenous diltiazem in acute myocardial infarction: Diltiazem as adjunctive therapy to activase (DATA) Trial. *J. Am. Coll. Cardiol.* 32:620–628, 1998.

Wilcox, R.G., Hampton, J.R., Banks, D.C., et al. Trial of early nifedipine in acute myocardial infarction: The Trent Study. *Br. Med. J.* 293:1204–1204, 1986.

Yusuf, S., Held, P., and Furberg, C. Update of effects of calcium antagonists in myocardial infarction or angina in light of the second Danish verapamil infarction trial (DAVIT-II) and other recent studies. *Am. J. Cardiol.* 67: 1295–1297, 1991.

17

Arrhythmias and their Treatment

All major forms of arrhythmias occur in the acutely ischemic myocardium. Standard textbooks should be employed to develop a fundamental understanding of the anatomy of the conduction system and the electrophysiologic principles of arrhythmias. Excellent examples of all the arrhythmias discussed in this chapter can be found in numerous textbooks. The following is an abbreviated approach to common rhythm disturbances in the setting of acute myocardial infarction (AMI).

SINUS BRADYCARDIA

Sinus bradycardia is a sinus mechanism with a ventricular rate of less than 60 beats per minute. It is a frequent accompaniment of AMI, particularly in the early phase of acute inferior infarction. There has been debate as to whether this rhythm affords a "protective" effect by raising the ventricular fibrillation threshold. Although this controversy has not yet been completely resolved, the final decision to treat sinus bradycardia must be based on the clinical judgment of the physician. In the absence of symptoms and when there are signs of good systemic perfusion, adequate blood pressure, and no significant ventricular arrhythmias, careful observation may be all that is required. If the heart rate consistently drops below 50 beats per minute or if the patient has signs of hypoperfusion, including chest pain, frequent premature ventricular contractions (PVCs), or low blood pressure, treatment should be instituted with intravenous atropine provided that no contraindications are present. The drug should be given by bolus in doses of 0.6 to 1.0 mg. Intravenous atropine in doses of 0.5 mg or less may sometimes paradoxically slow the heart by enhancing central nervous system parasympathetic outflow. If the heart rate does not increase in 2 to 4 minutes, the dose should be repeated. Should symptomatic bradycardia persist, a temporary pacemaker is preferable to other positive chronotropic measures (*chronotropic* means affecting the time or rate—i.e., the heart rate), such as an isoproterenol infusion, because pacing results in less oxygen demand. If atropine is initially successful, further doses should be repeated only if necessary, since repeated atropine usage may result in intolerable side

effects, including ileus, glaucomatous crisis, urinary retention, and, particularly in older patients, bizarre mental
behavior. If the drug has to be used on more than three
repeated occasions (such as every 2 to 4 hours), consideration should be given to the alternative treatment, temporary
pacing.

SINUS TACHYCARDIA

Sinus tachycardia is a sinus mechanism with a ventricular
rate greater than 100 beats per minute. The upper limit of
the rate is vague and varies according to age and physical
condition, but in adults it is usually considered to be 150
beats per minute. This is an extremely important arrhythmia in the coronary care unit (CCU) and can carry an ominous
prognosis, since myocardial oxygen consumption (MVO_2) is
linearly related to heart rate, and infarct size is related to
MVO_2 (see Chapter 12). This rhythm disturbance should be
aggressively investigated to see whether there is some treatable extracardiac or cardiac cause, such as residual chest
pain, infection, anxiety, pericarditis, or heart failure.

If there is no obvious explanation for the tachycardia and
the patient appears adequately sedated, it is possible that
the elevated heart rate is caused by hypovolemia or extensive MI. The latter differential can be very difficult, even for
the seasoned clinician. It may be important to resolve the
issue at once, since hypovolemia is correctable and sinus
tachycardia due to extensive myocardial necrosis implies a
poor prognosis. If the heart rate is persistently greater than
120 and the volume status is unclear, one should consider
measuring left-sided filling pressures with a flow-directed
catheter. Monitoring the central venous pressure (CVP) is
not a useful exercise in this setting, since right atrial pressure may be low despite elevated left atrial pressure, in
which case additional volume might precipitate pulmonary
edema. Moreover, the CVP may be elevated in patients with
cor pulmonale, secondary to chronic obstructive pulmonary
disease (COPD) in whom left-sided filling pressures are
often normal or low, and in whom the addition of a potent
diuretic could provoke hypotension. If the left-sided pressures are found to be low (<10 to 12 mm Hg), adding volume
to raise the pulmonary capillary wedge (PCW) pressure to
15 to 18 mm Hg will frequently correct the hypovolemia and
reduce the sinus tachycardia. If left-sided filling (wedge)
pressure is elevated (> 18 mm Hg), diuretic therapy may be
useful. Remember that both hypervolemia (elevated filling

pressure) and hypovolemia (low filling pressure) can increase MVO_2 and cause sinus tachycardia. These are unfavorable situations that can often be corrected, but the wrong choice of treatment (volume expansion versus diuretics) can provoke catastrophe (see also Chapter 19).

A small dose of beta-adenergic blocker may be useful in slowing sinus tachycardia provided that there is no pulmonary edema, shock, or other contraindication. Metoprolol (5 to 10 mg IV) can be used to slow persistent sinus tachycardia; but if stroke volume is low and cardiac output is marginal, hypotension can occur.

ATRIAL FIBRILLATION

In the large GUSTO-1 database, 2.5% of patients with AMI had atrial fibrillation on the admission electrocardiogram (ECG) and 7.9% developed atrial fibrillation after admission. These figures are in keeping with the previous experience that about 10% of patients with AMI have or develop atrial fibrillation. Patients with atrial fibrillation tend to have more three-vessel coronary artery disease and less than TIMI-3 coronary blood flow. In-hospital stroke is also significantly more common (3.1% of patients with atrial fibrillation versus 1.3% of patients with no atrial fibrillation). Patients with atrial fibrillation also tend to be older, have a worse Killip class, and have an increased heart rate on admission. The unadjusted mortality rate at 30 days is significantly higher (14.3% versus 6.2%), as it is at 1 year post-MI (21.5% versus 8.6%). The development of atrial fibrillation during the early phase of AMI carries a higher mortality, although much of the poor prognosis is due to confounding factors, such as advanced age and heart failure.

The primary therapy for atrial fibrillation that develops in the setting of AMI is direct current (DC) cardioversion (see Chapter 27). This is particularly important when the ventricular response is rapid, when there is hemodynamic compromise, or when there is associated myocardial ischemia. Patients with AMI who develop atrial fibrillation are usually already fully anticoagulated with heparin, and some will be receiving chronic warfarin. Transesophageal echocardiography can be performed when feasible to exclude intracardiac thrombi. Most cardiologists would prefer to do transesophageal echocardiography if the cardioversion is elective; in more urgent circumstances, however, transthoracic echocardiography may be sufficient. The presence of intracardiac thrombi, particularly if mobile, is a contraindication for electrical or chemical cardioversion, and long-term anti-coagulation and rate control is a more prudent strategy. In the absence of intra-cardiac thrombi, preparation for cardioversion should be considered, including consultation with anesthesiology. Patients should be anesthetized with 50 to 100 mg of methohexital sodium (Brevital) or 0.3 mg/kg of etomidate (Amidate). Synchronized DC cardioversion is performed using an initial shock of 200 J, because only 50% of patients can be converted with 100 J. About 85% of those who successfully cardiovert will do so at 200 J. The next shock should be 360 J, and this is successful in the vast majority of cases. If the first 360-J shock is not successful, one should wait a full 3 minutes before delivering a final 360-J shock. Systemic embolization occurs in 1% to 2% of all patients following DC cardioversion.

An occasional patient cannot be electrically cardioverted or has only temporary sinus rhythm and reverts quickly back to rapid atrial fibrillation. In such patients, the goal then becomes control of the ventricular rate with later conversion back to sinus rhythm. In such patients, heparin should be continued and intravenous amiodarone should be considered, as it will slow the ventricular rate (usually by 35 to 40 beats per minute in the first hour) and may actually increase the systolic blood pressure by about 25 mm Hg. The initial first-hour dose of amiodarone will depend on the patient's body weight and may vary from 60 mg over the first hour in a small patient to 1000 mg over 1 hour in a patient weighing 250 kg. A typical dose might be 5 mg/kg over 30 minutes followed by 1 mg/min over the ensuing 6 hours. After 6 hours, the infusion can be reduced to 0.5 mg/min to achieve a total loading dose of about 1200 mg over the first 24 hours. About 70% of patients will convert to normal sinus rhythm (NSR) by the end of the 24-hour period. In some patients hypotension may occur, but it can usually be ameliorated by slowing the rate of amiodarone infusion. After restoration of NSR, amiodarone can be continued orally at a low dose of 200 mg/day. Oral amiodorone is much less expensive than intravenous amiodarone. Even low-dose amiodarone is associated with a risk of toxicity and must be given in this setting for only a brief time (about 6 weeks). The risk of recurrent atrial fibrillation diminishes as time passes following MI.

For patients who are successfully cardioverted with DC countershock, an oral loading dose of amiodarone (10 mg/kg/day in two divided doses to reduce gastrointestinal complaints) can be started and continued for about 14 days. Following a cumulative oral loading dose of 6 g of amiodarone over 2 weeks, a maintenance dose of 200 mg/day can be started. A total duration of 6 weeks of amiodarone treatment may be sufficient, and the drug can then be stopped if NSR is restored. It is important to remember that amiodarone can interact with warfarin, and the intensity of the warfarin dose may have to be reduced to keep the International Normalized Ratio (INR) in the range of 2 to 3. Amiodarone also raises the digoxin level, requiring measurement of more frequent digoxin blood levels to avoid digoxin toxicity.

There are, of course, other, more time-honored methods than can be used to treat atrial fibrillation. However, atrial fibrillation in the setting of AMI is clearly a semi-urgent and serious complication. The rapid heart rate can drive myocardial oxygen demand, reduce filling time of the ventricle, and precipitate acute heart failure. DC cardioversion is the most direct and successful management strategy. Amiodarone is an excellent adjunctive therapy, and in some cases (e.g., failed DC cardioversion) becomes primary therapy. Although intravenous digoxin, procainamide, diltiazem, verapamil, ibutilide, and beta-adrenergic blockers can all slow the rapid ventricular response of atrial fibrillation, they are usually less effective than DC cardioversion or amiodarone in restoring NSR or may take longer to be effective. These drugs also frequently cause hypotension; in some cases, they are overtly pro-arrhythmic or poorly tolerated. Every case must be individualized, but DC cardioversion and amiodarone should at least be considered for all patients with the onset of rapid atrial fibrillation in the setting of AMI.

ATRIAL FLUTTER

Atrial flutter typically results in an atrial rate of between 280 and 320 beats per minute with a 2:1 A-V conduction ratio and a ventricular rate of about 150. It is occasionally seen in the setting of AMI (about 6%). Because of the rapid ventricular rate, cardioversion is the treatment of choice. The protocol for cardioversion is given in Chapter 27. Patients with atrial flutter should be anticoagulated, though the risk of systemic emboli with cardioversion is less than with atrial fibrillation. Atrial flutter is usually responsive to 25 to 50 J or less. When digitalis is used to manage atrial flutter, heroic doses are frequently required, time is lost, and cardioversion may still have to be resorted to later, often at greater risk because the patient has received large doses of digitalis. Atrial flutter may herald the onset of heart failure or shock and should alert the clinician to anticipate these complications.

SUPRAVENTRICULAR TACHYCARDIA

Rarely, supraventricular tachycardia (SVT) may provoke or complicate AMI. The rhythm is regular, with a rate between 160 and 300 (usually about 180) beats per minute. The ventricular response in SVT is usually faster than in sinus tachycardia and atrial flutter with block; it can be distinguished from ventricular tachycardia by its narrow QRS (unless there is associated aberrancy or bundle-branch block). Supraventricular tachycardia is most often transient and self-limited. Sustained SVT should be terminated immediately, even if there is no hemodynamic compromise, because the excessive heart rate leads to marked increases in MVO_2. Adenosine given as an intravenous bolus of 6 or 12 mg is now the treatment of choice for SVT. When this is given through a central line, only 3 mg is necessary. Mild side effects of brief duration include flushing, dyspnea, and chest discomfort.

Adenosine should not be used if patients are also receiving dipyramidole (which enhances its effects) or theophylline (which attenuates its effects). It can cause bronchoconstriction and should be avoided in patients with active airway obstruction, such as COPD or asthma. It may cause prolonged asystole in patients with sinus node dysfunction or in heart transplant patients. Intravenous verapamil (10 mg over 10 to 15 seconds with ECG and blood pressure monitoring) can also be given and repeated with carotid sinus massage, if necessary. Sometimes, electrical cardioversion is necessary. Usually 25 to 50 J will restore sinus rhythm. Termination of this arrhythmia with pressor agents, Valsalva maneuvers, and edrophonium is to be avoided in the setting of AMI. If SVT becomes recurrent and difficult to control, consultation with the electrophysiology (EP) service is indicated. Management can at times be difficult, and radiofrequency (RF) ablation may ultimately be necessary.

PREMATURE ATRIAL CONTRACTIONS

Premature atrial contractions (PACs) are common in AMI. The P waves have a different configuration from normal and may be peaked or inverted. They occur prematurely and result in an irregular rhythm. They are usually followed by a normal QRS but may not always conduct through to the ventricle (blocked PACs), particularly when they occur in the refractory period of the preceding QRS. They are frequently the result of heart failure, hypoxemia, or electrolyte disturbances and generally require no treatment. PACs are not infrequently the harbinger of atrial fibrillation.

WANDERING ATRIAL PACEMAKER
Wandering atrial pacemaker is due to P waves of varying ectopic origin (and of varying shape and position), resulting in a somewhat irregular rate. This arrhythmia should be approached in a manner similar to that for PACs.

PAROXYSMAL ATRIAL TACHYCARDIA WITH BLOCK
Paroxysmal atrial tachycardia (PAT) with block is unusual in the CCU. It is characterized by an atrial rate of 150 to 240 and usually results in a ventricular rate of about 110 to 120. The P waves are frequently smaller than usual and sometimes change shape. The differential diagnosis is usually between this rare arrhythmia and atrial flutter. Atrial flutter usually has larger P waves (frequently saw-toothed) and a faster ventricular rate (150). Digitalis toxicity is a common cause of PAT with block. In this setting, digitalis should be withheld and potassium salts administered, even if the serum potassium is normal. Cardioversion is contraindicated in PAT with block due to digitalis toxicity.

JUNCTIONAL RHYTHMS
Junctional rhythms are said to occur in 3% to 16% of patients with AMI. The incidence may be as high as 40% if computer-assisted continuous magnetic-tape recordings are used for detection. This arrhythmia originates within the bundle of His (the AV node has little or no actual pacemaker activity). The QRS complex is of normal duration, resembling the patient's normally conducted sinus beats. This rhythm may be slower than the normal sinus rate, in the range of 40 to 60 beats per minute, in which case it is a protective escape rhythm of no primary significance and should not be suppressed. If the ventricular response is extremely low or clinical deterioration occurs, one should consider atropine or pacemaker therapy or both. Occasionally, junctional beats occur as "extrasystoles," but they need not be as aggressively abolished. Digitalis excess, heart failure, hypokalemia, and hypoxemia should be considered as possible causes and corrected if present. Junctional rhythms sometimes begin abruptly with rates of 70 to 130 beats per minute (accelerated junctional rhythm). Such rhythm disturbances resemble supraventricular tachycardias, and if simple maneuvers such as carotid massage do not abort the

disturbance, cardioversion with low energy levels should be considered when the rate is rapid (heart rate > 120 beats per minute). Again, digitalis toxicity should be considered, and hypokalemia should be corrected.

MULTIFOCAL ATRIAL TACHYCARDIA

Multifocal atrial tachycardia (MAT), also known as chaotic atrial tachycardia, is not infrequently found in very seriously ill elderly patients, particularly when there is associated COPD or pneumonia. It is a manifestation of underlying disease and carries a poor prognosis. The ventricular rate may vary between 100 and 150 beats per minute. The atrial (and ventricular) rhythm is irregular because of varying P-R intervals and varying degrees of A-V block. The P waves vary in configuration with at least two ectopic foci. They are often peaked and tent-shaped, and the atrial rate may be extremely rapid, sometimes as high as 250 beats per minute. MAT may resemble ventricular tachycardia if there is associated QRS aberration or bundle-branch block. Multifocal atrial tachycardia is refractory to the usual treatment for supraventricular arrhythmias, and therapy directed to the underlying disease is more important than the administration of antiarrhythmic drugs. Heart failure, pH and electrolyte imbalance, and hypoxemia should be corrected. Cardioversion entails some risk and is generally not successful. Small doses of an intravenous beta-adrenergic blocking drug may occasionally be successful in slowing the ventricular rate, but such drugs should be avoided in patients with COPD, decompensated heart failure, or both.

ATRIOVENTRICULAR DISSOCIATION

The term *atrioventricular* (A-V) *dissociation* refers to a group of arrhythmias in which the atria and ventricles beat independently, so that the P waves and the QRS complexes have no certain relationship. This condition is seen in complete A-V block, ventricular tachycardia, and various supraventricular arrhythmias. The treatment obviously depends on the underlying cardiac mechanism, the ventricular rate, and the patient's condition.

PREMATURE VENTRICULAR CONTRACTIONS

Also called *ventricular premature beats,* premature ventricular contractions (PVCs) are omnipresent in patients who have sustained an acute MI and sometimes predict the onset of more serious ventricular arrhythmias. They are characterized by a widened, bizarre QRS with abnormal-appearing T waves occurring early in the cardiac cycle without any meaningful relationship to the preceding P wave. Ventricular escape beats and rhythms that occur in the setting of A-V block should be considered separately.

In CCUs with continuous monitoring, PVCs have been noticed in almost all patients with AMI if their heart rhythm is recorded for at least 24 hours empirically. Physiologists and clinicians have also long been aware that the coupling interval between the preceding beat and the PVC (i.e., the degree of PVC prematurity) has arrhythmogenic significance. When the R wave of the PVC falls on the T wave of the preceding beat, ventricular tachycardia or fibrillation may be provoked. This "R on T" phenomenon was once considered an indication for antiarrhythmic therapy. More recent studies have indicated that the malignancy of a ventricular ectopic beat may not necessarily be determined by its coupling interval or its configuration. Moreover, ventricular tachycardia and ventricular fibrillation are usually not preceded by these so-called warning arrhythmias.

It is important, of course, to remember that PVCs in the presence of AMI may not always be due to ischemia. Hypokalemia and heart failure can provoke ventricular arrhythmias and must be treated. Attention should be paid to anxiety and hypoxemia. Occasionally, the presence of CVP lines or a Swan-Ganz catheter will provoke PVCs and atrial arrhythmias. The PVCs usually take the configuration of left bundle-branch block in these cases, since they are generated from the right ventricle. Usually this situation is easily corrected by repositioning the catheter.

Experience in CCUs over the past 40 years has repeatedly confirmed that frequent and complex PVCs can culminate in ventricular tachycardia and ventricular fibrillation (VF). At one time prophylactic suppression of PVCs by intravenous lidocaine was the cornerstone of therapy in the CCU. The issue of the safety and efficacy of prophylactic lidocaine in this context has recently been re-examined, and there appears to be a trend for increased mortality in lidocaine-treated patients, possibly due to excess fatal bradycardia or asystolic arrests. The routine use of prophylactic lidocaine should probably be avoided. Primary VF may be declining, even if one corrects for the use of prophylactic lidocaine. It has been estimated that 400 patients must be treated with prophylactic lidocaine to prevent one episode of VF. Presumably, the more widespread use of thrombolytic therapy, beta-adrenergic blockers, aspirin, and heparin means that early anti-ischemic therapy is now more intense than in the past. Less acute ischemia means fewer cases of VF. Given the well-known toxicity of lidocaine, the use of prophylactic lidocaine should now be discouraged. The use of lidocaine for frequent or complex PVCs has also diminished considerably in recent years.

When the decision is made to consider using lidocaine, many factors such as age and hepatic function must be carefully considered. In averaged-sized patients with presumably normal cardiac output and normal hepatic function, a loading dose should be administered aimed at delivering 200 mg over a 10-to 12-minute period. This can be achieved by giving a 100-mg bolus over 2 minutes and repeating this dose 10 minutes later. Alternatively, a 50-mg dose can be given at 1 minute and repeated four times at 5-minute intervals; or 20 mg/min may be infused for 10 minutes. Following this, a continuous dose using an infusion-regulating device should be delivered at 2 to 4 mg/min for 24 to 30 hours (average dose, 3 mg/min). To raise the plasma concentration acutely (for arrhythmia breakthrough), a 50-mg bolus should be given over 1 minute, and the infusion rate should simultaneously be increased to no more than 4 mg/min. In shock, heart failure, and hepatocellular disease as well as in patients over 70 years of age, the loading dose and the rate of maintenance infusion should be reduced by half and the serum concentration of lidocaine should be monitored frequently (daily or more often if toxicity is suspected). The therapeutic plasma lidocaine level varies from 1.4 to 6.0 µg/ml.

Because of the marked fat solubility of the drug, it takes several hours to produce a new steady-state blood level of lidocaine by simply increasing the continuous infusion rate. This is why patients need to be re-bolused. Similarly, when a decision is made to discontinue lidocaine, weaning is not necessary; simply stopping the infusion will suffice. Patients with PVCs resistant to lidocaine are not rare (approximately 20%), but other causes (such as infiltrated intravenous lines) should be sought before using the maximal continuous infusion rate of 4 mg/min.

Lidocaine is metabolized in the liver, and agents or block that induce hepatic enzymes may alter lidocaine metabolism. Cimetidine can promote lidocaine toxicity. Serious toxic side effects include focal and grand mal seizures, psychosis, and, rarely, respiratory arrest. Paresthesias, muscle twitching, disorientation, drowsiness, and hearing loss may occur and may necessitate reducing or stopping the drug. Convulsions respond to intravenous diazepam or barbiturates; frequently, stopping the infusion will ameliorate the seizure.

Lidocaine appears to have minimal negative inotropic effects (*inotropic* means affecting the force of contraction); heart rate, blood pressure, and cardiac output do not change significantly unless very large doses are given. Additionally, the drug ordinarily has little or no effect on the conduction system and can usually be administered safely in the presence of conduction disturbances. Occasionally, lidocaine suppresses sinus node activity, and severe bradycardia can ensue. The threshold response to artificial pacing is not changed by lidocaine.

Intravenous procainamide is also effective against PVCs in AMI, and it is a relatively safe alternative to lidocaine (see Appendix I). However, like lidocaine, it is rarely used to simply suppress PVCs in the current era. It can be employed together with lidocaine to suppress sustained ventricular ectopic activity refractory to either drug alone. The oral absorption of procainamide may be erratic in the early hours after MI, and parenteral drug administration is preferred in this setting. A loading dose of 10 to 12 mg/kg should be given intravenously at a rate that does not exceed 25 mg/min. For most patients, this dose is given over 30 to 40 minutes. Blood pressure, ECG, and clinical status must be monitored continuously, because hypotension and arrhythmias may occur. If a continuous infusion is required, the usual rate is 2 mg/min. Although the average patient requires 50 mg/kg/day as a maintenance dose, there can be wide variation, and the dose should be based on the plasma concentration of the drug. The effective plasma concentration using intravenous procainamide is 4 to 8 µg/ml, which appears to result in no significant alteration in hemodynamic function. The drug causes minimal prolongation of A-V conduction time but significant prolongation of His-Purkinje conduction time, and should therefore be used with caution in patients with impaired conduction systems (bundle branch block or ventricular conduction delay) unless an artificial pacemaker is in place. Procainamide can also increase the threshold response to artificial pacing and may result in failure of the pacemaker to initiate a ventricular depolarization.

It has been suggested that lidocaine is more effective than procainamide in preventing ventricular re-entrant activity induced by early premature beats. Re-entry, which is characterized by closely coupled beats with fixed coupling intervals, results from depressed conductivity in an ischemic area of the ventricle. PVCs due to increased automaticity of the Purkinje tissue of the ventricle appear to be less likely to provoke ventricular tachycardia and fibrillation. The distinction between the two mechanisms is not always clear on the scalar tracing. Despite similarities in the elctrophysiologic properties of certain antiarrhythmic drugs, it is possible for ventricular irritability that cannot be suppressed by one antiarrhythmic agent (e.g., procainamide) to be suppressed by another antiarrhythmic drug with the same elctrophysiological properties (e.g., quinidine). The plasma half-life of procainamide is about 3 1/2 hours (longer in the sustained action form), and the drug should be stopped if the QRS is prolonged by more than 50%. The kidneys are responsible for most of its elimination, and the half-life is prolonged when there is renal impairment. The drug is often poorly tolerated when administered orally for more than a few days.

Although it has been suggested that *N*-acetyl-procainamide (NAPA) is an active antiarrhythmic metabolite of procainamide, most patients probably do not achieve plasma concentrations of NAPA high enough to result in important antiarrhythmic activity. Antinuclear antibodies will develop in at least half the patients receiving long-term procainamide therapy; in approximately 20% of these patients, some form of clinical systemic lupus erythematosus will develop. The drug-induced syndrome is distinguished from systemic lupus erythematosus by the absence of renal involvement, and it is abolished by discontinuing the drug.

Occasionally, PVCs may occur with AMI due to the mechanism of parasystole. This mechanism is identified by varying coupling intervals in which the inter-ectopic intervals are equal to a multiple of the shortest inter-ectopic interval. Long rhythm strips are sometimes needed to make this diagnosis. The arrhythmia usually arises from an independent ventricular pacemaker and does not ordinarily deteriorate into sustained ventricular tachyarrhythmias. It responds less well to antiarrhythmic therapy than do other arrhythmias, and aggressive treatment may lead to lidocaine toxicity. In fact, treatment of this arrhythmia may be unnecessary.

SUSTAINED VENTRICULAR TACHYCARDIA

Ventricular tachycardia (VT) is conventionally described as a sequence of three or more ventricular extrasystoles at rates ranging from 100 to 250/min. Sustained VT culminating in symptoms is a serious complication of AMI and may require cardioversion and drug therapy (e.g., lidocaine or amiodarone). It is frequently seen during AMI (16% to 40%), and its occurrence is favored by large infarctions and heart failure. The mechanism of VT at one time was ascribed to an accelerated discharge from a single ventricular ectopic focus, but it is now believed that many episodes of VT with acute MI are due to re-entry. When the rate of VT is less than 100 (this figure being used somewhat arbitrarily), the rhythm is usually considered an accelerated idioventricular rhythm and takes on a different connotation; when the VT rate exceeds 250 beats per minute, it is best to consider the rhythm ventricular flutter. Most episodes of VT have considerable regularity, with minimal beat-to-beat variation. There is more irregularity when the arrhythmia begins or is terminated, and variation in regularity is also more common in accelerated idioventricular rhythm. Cardiac function is usually compromised, although beats generated from the apex of the left ventricle maybe more hemodynamically effective than are beats arising from basilar areas of the heart. Any signs of A-V dissociation, such as fusion or capture beats, are of diagnostic aid in identifying VT. Atrioventricular dissociation can result in wide splitting of the first and second heart sounds, variable intensity of the first heart sound, and intermittent cannon "a" waves in the jugular pulse. Carotid sinus massage is usually ineffective in slowing the ventricular rate. The diagnosis of VT is further supported when the QRS complexes have a morphology similar to those of the patient's preexisting PVCs. A left axis deviation and Q/S ratio > 1 in V_6 also favor VT.

Diagnostic maneuvers should not delay treatment for this life-threatening arrhythmia. If the patient is unconscious or in shock, a thump to the precordium followed by electrical DC cardioversion (when sinus rhythm is not restored) is recommended. Rapid, polymorphic VT should be treated with an unsynchronized discharge of 200 J, while monomorphic VT with rates >150 beats per minute can be treated with a 100-J synchronized discharge. If the patient is otherwise stable, a brief trial of an antiarrhythmic agent is warranted as a first approach.

Sustained ventricular tachycardia that is well tolerated by the patient and does not compromise the circulation can be treated with intravenous lidocaine (50- to 100-mg bolus, repeated in 2 minutes if the rhythm is not abolished) or intravenous amiodarone. Amiodarone may be more effective and less toxic. As with atrial fibrillation, intravenous amiodarone should be given as a loading dose (5 mg/kg over 30 minutes), and this is followed by an infusion of 1 mg/min for the next 6 hours. After 6 hours, the amiodarone dose can be reduced to 0.5 mg/h to achieve a total loading dose of ~ 1200 mg over 24 hours. After a cumulative loading dose of 6 g has been given, an oral dose of 200 to 400 mg/day can be used to control further arrhythmias. Patients with recurrent sustained VT should have coronary angiography followed by an EP consult. In some cases they may benefit from reperfusion therapy, an EP study, or an automatic implantable cardioverter defibrillator (AICD).

A specific type of VT called *torsades de pointes* can occur in patients with a long QT interval. The rhythm appears to be twisting on its axis (polymorphic) or iso-electric line. Torsades de pointes is best treated with 2 g of intravenous magnesium sulfate (bolus) followed by 3 to 20 mg/min until the QT interval is less than 0.50 seconds. Occasionally, overdrive pacing or isoproterenol is necessary.

When pharmacologic therapy fails to control recurrent VT, bursts of rapid ventricular pacing should be considered as an alternative method of treatment. This is particularly important if repeated external DC shocks are necessary (a situation one wishes to avoid). Ventricular tachycardia has been terminated by pacing at rates just in excess of the ventricular rate and then slowly decreasing the pacing rate (entertainment). Random or programmed extrasystoles may also terminate VT, but this requires skilled adjustments by the operator of the pacemaker. Bursts of rapid ventricular pacing appear to be a benign and effective mode of therapy for recurrent VT and are simpler to manage than is programmed stimulation. There is no discomfort to the patient, and this therapy may be used numerous times without the physical and psychological stress of DC cardioversion. Ventricular fibrillation may be precipitated by this technique, and VT may be accelerated. The advantages appear to outweigh the risks in severe cases; however, and the method appears to be a useful addition to other therapies for recurrent VT until a more permanent form of treatment such as reperfusion of an acid or radiofrequency ablation can be applied.

ACCELERATED IDIOVENTRICULAR RHYTHM

Accelerated idioventricular rhythm (AIVR) is an interesting and somewhat controversial arrhythmia known by a wide variety of names (frequently it is referred to incorrectly as *slow ventricular tachycardia*). Although it is seen in many different heart conditions as well as in cases of digitalis intoxication, it is not rare (13% to 30%) during the first 48 hours of AMI, particularly in inferior MIs. AIVR today is most commonly the result of reperfusion of an occluded coronary artery, either spontaneous or due to thrombolytic therapy. It is usually non-sustained, well tolerated by the patient, and rarely requires any treatment. It is characterized by three or more widened QRS complexes occurring at a rate similar to the prevailing sinus rate and may alternate with periods of sinus rhythm. The first beat of a paroxysm tends to occur during the slow phase of sinus arrhythmia and has a long coupling interval to the preceding beat. It nearly always occurs at a rate of less than 100 and should not technically be considered a tachycardia. Dissociated P waves can be seen in the majority of cases of AIVR, and the beats are not preceded by His deflections on His bundle electrograms. This confirms the supposition that AIVR is not supraventricular in origin.

A benign course has been observed in cases of AIVR, and the usual teaching has been not to suppress these beats if the patient is otherwise stable. In fact, some authors believe that treatment may be contraindicated, since suppression of what may be an "escape" mechanism can result in asystole. However, other authorities believe the arrhythmia is due to an ectopic focus with intermittent exit block. If the arrhythmia results in a slow ventricular rate with attendant problems such as hypotension or other signs of hypoperfusion (which in part may be due to loss of "atrial kick"), treatment with atropine (0.6 to 1.0 mg IV) is recommended provided that there are no contraindications. Atropine increases the sinus rate, thus overdriving the ectopic focus. If atropine is contraindicated or fails to abolish the rhythm, an artificial transvenous pacemaker should be considered. Currently, the treatment of sustained AIVR remains controversial and rests in large part on the physician's judgment.

BIDIRECTIONAL VENTRICULAR TACHYCARDIA

Bidirectional ventricular tachycardia (VT) is an uncommon arrhythmia characterized by QRS complexes with a right bundle-branch block pattern in the frontal plane and an alternative morphology (seen only in the limb leads) an upward complex in one beat and a downward complex in the next. The rate is between 140 and 180 in most cases; the QRS is widened, with an axis in the frontal plane alternating between −60 to −80° and + 120°. Bidirectional VT is most often seen in the setting of digitalis intoxication, but it can occur in AMI. The ectopic focus is probably ventricular, since the complexes are not preceded by a His spike during His ECGs. The rhythm can be abolished with intravenous lidocaine.

VENTRICULAR FIBRILLATION

Ventricular fibrillation (VF) is easily recognized by its chaotic, undulating morphology, which is due to wandering of the cardiac impulse continuously along constantly changing pathways. This results in fully contracting fibers and fully relaxed fibers at the same time. When it occurs in an organized, coarse fashion, it may spontaneously revert to a less primitive rhythm, but this is rare, and immediate cardioversion is nearly always indicated. When a patient is found pulseless on the ward in a non-monitored state and rhythm is not clear, so-called blind defibrillation should be performed because of the high probability that VF or VT is present. Only about 20% of cardiac arrests in the CCU are due to "straight-line" asystole, 75% being due to VF. This recommendation (i.e., blind defibrillation) is supported by the well-known fact that the time delay provoked by such measures as applying ECG leads and attempting intubation prior to defibrillation greatly lessens the chance of establishing an effective rhythm.

For patients weighing more than 50 kg, 200 to 300 J should be used. Repeated, frequent attempts at defibrillation with 400 J may cause myocardial damage. Primary VF occurred in about 10% of patients with AMI at one time. The incidence has seemingly decreased in recent years. About 50% of episodes of VF occur within 4 hours of the onset of acute MI, and 80% occur in the first 12 hours. The prognosis of patients who develop primary VF is still debated. There may be excessive in-hospital mortality, but late mortality is not much affected by early primary VF.

Patients resuscitated from out-of-hospital cardiac arrest who survive hospitalization and have no obvious AMI are becoming increasingly more common because of the emergency medical rescue teams operating in large cities. Long-term follow-up of such patients has identified them as a group at high risk of recurrent VF and sudden death. Studies have indicated that most of these patients will continue to have chronic asymptomatic complex ventricular arrhythmias that are often resistant to various antiarrhythmic regimens. Ventricular fibrillation that occurs outside the setting of AMI is associated with a much worse prognosis than VF that occurs during AMI. The management of this difficult problem is still evolving. In general, patients with VF and no AMI should undergo diagnostic coronary angiography and should have an EP study. Treatment often consists of reperfusion therapy, an AICD, and amiodarone. The prognosis is determined by the extent of LV dysfunction and amount of underlying coronary artery disease.

VENTRICULAR ARRHYTHMIAS IN THE LATE HOSPITAL PHASE OF ACUTE MYOCARDIAL INFARCTION

When arrhythmias abate early after AMI, long-term antiarrhythmic therapy after discharge is not necessary. Several studies have indicated, however, that complex and frequent ventricular ectopy may persist in the late hospital period and after discharge. Moreover, these arrhythmias make an independent contribution to the increased persistent risk of death. For this and other reasons, it is desirable to continue to monitor patients by telemetry when they leave the CCU. Personnel in the "intermediate cardiac unit" should be familiar with cardiopulmonary resuscitation techniques and arrhythmia surveillance. It appears as though the prevalence of complex and frequent arrhythmias may be linked to the extent of left ventricular dysfunction. Information from the Cardiac Arrhythmia Suppression Trial (CAST) indicates that several antiarrhythmic drugs may worsen survival through their proarrhythmic properties. Patients with symptomatic ventricular arrhythmias, sustained ventricular tachycardia, or late primary VF should be referred to an electrophysiologist for invasive electrophysiology studies to determine effective therapy. In many cases, this will include an AICD plus therapy with an antiarrhythmic drug such as amiodarone.

PROTOCOL

1. Sinus bradycardia:
   a. No treatment if the patient is stable.
   b. Heart rate well below 50 beats per minute, particularly when associated with chest pain, PVCs, or hypotension, should be treated with intravenous boluses of atropine (0.6 to 1.0 mg).
   c. If atropine is contraindicated, fails to increase the heart rate, or has to be employed more than three times in 6 to 12 hours, placement of a temporary pacing catheter should be considered.
2. Sinus tachycardia:
   d. Define the underlying etiology: infection, anxiety, pericarditis, hypovolemia, left ventricular failure, pain.

   b. Catheterization of the pulmonary artery should be considered. If the PCW pressure is low (< 10 mm Hg), volume expansion (e.g., saline, plasma, salt-poor albumin, dextran) is useful. If PCW pressure is elevated (>18 mm Hg), intravenous furosemide should be given.
   c. If PCW and cardiac output are normal, intravenous metoprolol (10 to 15 mg) should be considered.
3. Atrial fibrillation:
   a. DC cardioversion for patients with hemodynamic compromise or myocardial ischemia.
   b. IV amiodarone (5 mg/kg over 30 minutes followed by 1 mg/min for the next 6 hours; then 0.5 mg/min until a total dose of ~ 1200 mg over 24 hours is given; infusion of 0.5 to 1 mg/min can be continued or patient can be switched to an oral dose of 200 mg per day to maintain NSR).
   c. Heparin.
   d. Rapid digitalization or IV beta-blockers (if not contraindicated) to slow the ventricular rate.
4. Atrial flutter: cardioversion is the preferred treatment of this arrhythmia, since it is frequently difficult to control the ventricular response with digitalis.
5. Supraventricular tachycardia:
   a. Sustained SVT should be treated with intravenous adenosine if the SVT does not abort easily with carotid massage. DC cardioversion may be necessary. The use of pressor agents, Valsalva maneuvers, and edrophonium should be avoided in acute MI.
6. Premature atrial contractions: other than definition of their etiology (frequently, heart failure), no therapy is required for PACs.
7. Wandering atrial pacemaker: these arrhythmias are treated in a manner similar to that for PACs.
8. Paroxysmal atrial tachycardia with block:
   a. Digitalis intoxication should be strongly considered.
   b. Serum K^+ should be monitored and potassium chloride (KCL) administered if a low-normal serum K^+ value is obtained.
   c. Cardioversion should not be attempted if digitalis intoxication is suspected.
9. Junctional rhythms:
   a. Slow junctional rhythm is usually a protective escape mechanism; as such, it need not be treated

as long as the ventricular rate is adequate. If the ventricular response is extremely slow or clinical deterioration occurs, atropine, pacemaker therapy, or both [analogous to sinus bradycardia (see page 99)] should be considered.

b. Rapid and sustained junctional tachycardia should be treated in a manner similar to that for SVT: carotid massage followed by cardioversion unless digitalis toxicity is suspected.

10. Multifocal atrial tachycardia: this arrhythmia is frequently difficult to abort. It is essential to treat the underlying pulmonary and metabolic problems. Cardioversion and digitalis therapy are not usually indicated.

11. Atrioventricular dissociation: the treatment of this rhythm disturbance depends on its cause. When the ventricular rate is adequate and the patient is stable, no therapy is necessary.

12. Premature ventricular contractions and ventricular tachycardia:

a. No treatment necessary for asymptomatic PVCs or non-sustained VT.

b. Consider IV amiodarone for sustained VT if patient is stable; if patient is unstable, use DC cardioversion.

c. Rarely, IV lidocaine 200-mg bolus over 10 to 20 minutes followed by infusion of 2 to 4 mg/min. Use only for sustained VT; IV amiodarone may be safer and more effective but is more expensive.

13. Accelerated idioventricular rhythm:

a. The questions of what kind of treatment and even whether or not to treat are controversial. If the patient is stable, no treatment is necessary. This arrhythmia may be a sign of reperfusion.

b. If the patient is deteriorating, the rhythm may be overdriven by means of intravenous atropine (0.6 to 1.0 mg) or suppressed by intravenous lidocaine (50- to 200-mg IV bolus, followed by an infusion of 204 mg/min).

14. Ventricular fibrillation:

a. Immediate cardioversion with 200 to 300 J is essential. If reversion to sinus rhythm does not occur, closed-chest cardiac massage, endotracheal intubation, and intravenous bicarbonate should be administered, followed by repeated attempts at cardioversion.

BIBLIOGRAPHY

Antman, E.M., and Berlin, J.A. Declining incidence of ventricular fibrillation in myocardial infarction: Implications for the prophylactic use of lidocaine. *Circulation* 86: 764–773, 1992.

The Cardiac Arrhythmia Suppression Trial (CAST) Investigators. Increased mortality due to encainide or flecainide in a randomized trial of arrhythmia suppression after myocardial infarction. *N. Engl. J. Med.* 321:406–412, 1989.

Chiribota, D., Yarzebski, J., Goldberg, R.J., Gore, J.M., and Alpert, J.S. Temporal trends (1975 through 1990) in the incidence and case-fatality rates of primary ventricular fibrillation complicating acute myocardial infarction. *Circulation* 89:998–1003, 1994.

Clemo, H.F., Wood, M.A., Gilligan, D.M., and Ellenbogen, K.A. Intravenous amiodarone for acute heart rate control in the critically ill patient with atrial tachyarrhythmias. *Am. J. Cardiol.* 81:594–598, 1998.

Crenshaw, B.S., Ward, S.R., Granger, C.B., et al. Atrial fibrillation in the setting of acute myocardial infarction: The GUSTO-I experience. *J. Am. Coll. Cardiol.* 30:406–413, 1997.

Eldar, M., Canetti, M., Rotstein, Z., et al. Significance of paroxysmal atrial fibrillation complicating acute myocardial infarction in thrombolytic era. *Circulation* 97: 965–970, 1998.

Kowey, P.R., Marinchak, R.A., Rials, S.J., and Filart, R. A. Intravenous amiodarone. *J. Am. Coll. Cardiol.* 29: 1190–1198, 1997.

Opolski, G., Stanislawska, J., Gorecki, A., Swiecicka, G., Torbicki, A., and Kraska, T. Amiodarone in restoration and maintenance of sinus rhythm in patients with chronic atrial fibrillation after unsuccessful direct-current cardioversion. *Clin. Cardiol.* 20:337–340, 1997.

Roy, D., Talajic, M., Thibault, B., et al. Pilot study and protocol of the Canadian trial of atrial fibrillation (CTAF). *Am. J. Cardiol.* 80:464–468, 1997.

Sakata, K., Kurihara, H., Iwamori, K., et al. Clinical and prognostic significance of atrial fibrillation in acute myocardial infarction. *Am. J. Cardiol.* 80:1522–1527, 1997.

Shen, W.K., and Hammill, S.C. Survivors of acute myocardial infarction: Who is at risk for sudden death? *Mayo Clin. Proc.* 66:950–962, 1991.

Singh, B. N. Routine prophylactic lidocaine administration in acute myocardial infarction: An idea whose time is all but gone? *Circulation* 86:1033–1035, 1992.

Stevenson, W.G., and Ridker, P.M. Should survivors of myocardial infarction with low ejection fraction be routinely referred to arrhythmia specialist? *J.A.M.A.* 276: 481–485, 1996.

Wolfe, C.L., Nibley, C., Bhandari, A., Chatterjee, K., and Scheinman, M. Polymorphous ventricular tachycardia associated with acute myocardial infarction. *Circulation* 84:1543–1551, 1991.

18

Pacemakers: Indications for and Technique of Insertion

There is still considerable uncertainty and variable opinion regarding the indications for temporary pacing in the setting of acute myocardial infarction (AMI). This is because there are no randomized, controlled trials to help guide physicians in the management of transient conduction disturbances secondary to AMI. The criteria for insertion of temporary pacemakers for A-V block related to AMI, unlike those for permanent pacing, do not necessarily depend on the presence of symptoms. The indications for pacing in the setting of AMI are primarily related to the presence of intraventricular conduction defects. The reported incidence and significance of various conduction disturbances varies widely in the literature. In the thrombolytic era, which has diminished the incidence of A-V block in AMI, the mortality has remained high when A-V block occurs. The long-term prognosis of patients with AMI who develop A-V block is primarily related to the extent of myocardial damage rather than to the A-V block itself. When intraventricular conduction abnormalities occur in the setting of AMI, with the exception of isolated left anterior fascicular block, there is an unfavorable short- and long-term prognosis and increased incidence of sudden death. The poor prognosis is often related to associated extensive myocardial damage and is not necessarily due to the A-V block itself.

The nature of the A-V block and the location of the infarct are also important. A-V block that develops during the course of an inferior MI can be associated with a favorable long-term outcome, although in-hospital survival is impaired. Patients who develop conduction abnormalities with an anterior MI have a somewhat worse prognosis. Pacemakers should not be implanted if the A-V block is expected to resolve and the patient is tolerating the conduction disturbance well, as is often the case in patients with inferior MI.

Patients with acute inferior MI frequently have sinus bradycardia, particularly within the first hour. Sinus bradycardia also occurs with other forms of MI and is often the result of increased parasympathetic activity. About 30% to 40% of patients with AMI develop sinus bradycardia. Interventricular conduction delays are reported to occur in 10% to 20% of patients with AMI. The risk of developing complete heart block in the setting of AMI is increased if the patient demonstrates first-degree A-V block, Mobitz type I A-V block, Mobitz type II A-V block, left anterior fascicular block, left posterior fascicular block, right bundle-branch block and left bundle-branch block.

SINUS NODE DYSFUNCTION

The diagnosis of sinus or atrial standstill is established by the sudden loss of atrial activity in the electrocardiogram (ECG). It is unclear how often this occurs with AMI, but it is more likely to be seen if the patient has the so-called sick-sinus syndrome, in which both atrial tachyarrhythmias and marked sinus bradycardia may occur. Rarely, sinus arrest will be precipitated by certain drugs, including lidocaine and H_2 (histamine) blockers. *Sinoatrial exit block* is suspected when the pause is a multiple of the spontaneous sinus cycle length. A pause that is not a multiple of the underlying sinus cycle length is referred to as a *sinus pause;* it is called a *sinus arrest* when it is very prolonged. The period of asystole rarely lasts more than 5 to 10 seconds and is usually terminated by atrial or junctional complexes. Pauses greater than 3 to 4 seconds, particularly when recurrent, usually require temporary pacing. Often, one or more blows to the lower sternum may rapidly restore sinus rhythm. Emergency therapy for prolonged or repeated sinus arrest includes the use of intravenous atropine (0.6 to 1.0 mg). This drug may not be successful, however, unless increased vagal tone is the mechanism of the abnormality. Infusion of intravenous isoproterenol HCl (1 mg in 250 mg of 5% D/W) may be helpful in enhancing sinus node activity and will often result in a ventricular escape rate adequate for perfusion during an emergency. Use of a temporary transvenous ventricular pacemaker is the only way of ensuring that repeated episodes of serious bradycardia do not occur.

ATRIOVENTRICULAR BLOCK

When bradycardia due to A-V block occurs in the setting of AMI, it is important to localize the site of infarction. With inferior MI, the occurrence of A-V block is usually heralded by a progressive prolongation of the P-R interval (first-degree A-V block). This is followed by second-degree A-V block of the Wenckebach type, which is characterized by nonconducted sinus impulses preceded by progressive prolongation of the P-R interval. Patients who develop the Wenckebach phenomenon are generally not candidates for a pacemaker. This form of A-V block is usually a temporary event related to ischemia or edema of the A-V node or due to excessive vagal tone. Such patients should be carefully observed for signs of adequate perfusion, including a close check of the blood pressure, mental status, urine output, and so on. The Wenckebach phenomenon tends to resolve in 24 to 48 hours, but it may occasionally persist for several days.

Patients who develop Mobitz type II conduction disturbance (characterized by a constant P-R interval despite dropped beats) with a wide QRS complex and slow ventricular rate—particularly if associated with anterior MI, fascicular block, or bundle-branch block—are candidates for a temporary pacemaker. Such patients usually have permanent damage to part of the conduction system and often proceed to complete heart block (CHB), sometimes suddenly.

When 2:1 AV block develops during AMI, the actual site of the conduction disturbance cannot be clearly ascertained by the scalar ECG. The decision to pace temporarily will depend on the judgment of the physician: the patient with an inferior MI and a narrow QRS, adequate ventricular rate, and no signs or symptoms of hypoperfusion may sometimes be observed without a pacemaker. Pacing may become necessary if the patient develops hypotension, or chest pain or shows other signs of inadequate perfusion.

Sudden CHB usually occurs because of failure of impulse conduction through the His-Purkinje system. The resultant bradycardia is usually profound. The ECG shows no relationship of P waves to the QRS, and the ventricular complex is usually wide and slow. Emergency treatment consists of giving isoproterenol HCl to increase the rate of the idioventricular pacemaker (a starting dose of 1 μg/min can be used by infusing a solution of 1 mg in 250 ml of 5% D/W administered at a rate of 0.25 ml/min). Occasionally, a large dose of atropine is effective. Plans should immediately be made for insertion of a temporary transvenous ventricular pacemaker.

FASCICULAR AND BUNDLE-BRANCH BLOCK

It is estimated that 15% to 20% of patients with AMI will develop fascicular or bundle-branch block. The hospital mortality of this complication may range up to 50%, in part because these conduction disturbances are often associated with severe pump failure. Isolated left anterior fascicular block and left posterior fascicular block are unusual (5% and 1%, respectively); because they rarely progress to complete A-V block (0 to 3%), they do not require placement of a prophylactic temporary pacemaker. The development of right bundle-branch block plus left anterior fascicular block is rare (1% of AMI patients), but also frequently progresses to complete heart block and requires placement of a temporary pacemaker. Left bundle-branch block develops in about 0.5% of patients with AMI, and although it progresses to complete A-V block less commonly (20%), it probably should be considered a potential indication for placement of a temporary pacemaker. The development of isolated right bundle-branch block occurs in about 2% of patients but progresses to high-grade A-V block in 40% to 45% of cases and therefore should also be considered a potential indication for standby pacing. There is still considerable uncertainty, however, regarding the need for pacing in right bundle-branch block and left bundle-branch block in the setting of AMI. Associated first-degree A-V block appears to add to the risk of developing complete A-V block. The prognostic significance of preexisting bundle-branch block in patients with AMI is likewise an unsettled issue. In our opinion, the failure of published reports to demonstrate improved prognosis statistically does not offset the value of pacemaker therapy in individual patients. The generally poor prognosis associated with these conduction disorders is more reflective of extensive underlying infarction than of progression of A-V block. Nonetheless, the use of standby temporary pacemakers will undoubtedly continue to save individual lives of high-risk patients.

The large number of risk variables, plus the conflicting data reported for each individual risk variable, present the clinician with a bewildering array of suggestions and make the decision regarding placement of a temporary pacemaker extremely difficult. One possible way to deal with the dilemma is to assign a risk score of 1 to each well-recognized type of conduction disorder (first-degree A-V block, Mobitz type II block, CHB, left anterior fascicular block, left posterior fascicular block, complete left bundle-branch block, complete right bundle-branch block). Scores of 0, 1, 2, or 3 or more are associated with incidences of CHB of 1.2, 7.8, 25, and 35.4%, respectively. Patients with a risk score of 2 demonstrate an intermediate risk of developing CHB. Those patients with a risk score of 2 or more and an anterior MI should undergo prophylactic temporary transvenous pacing. Patients with an inferior MI and a risk score of 2 are well suited for the prophylactic use of an external noninvasive cardiac pacemaker, as described by Zoll and colleagues. Temporary transvenous pacing probably improves survival in only a small fraction of patients—for example, patients with complete A-V block and anterior wall infarction.

PERMANENT PACEMAKERS

Certain patients appear to benefit from permanent pacing before discharge from the hospital. Those who develop acute bifascicular block associated with high-grade A-V block (Mobitz type II or CHB) sometime during their hospital stay should be considered for this therapy. All patients who progress to high-grade A-V block during the course of infarction, irrespective of the site of infarction or whether normal A-V conduction returns, should be considered for a permanent pacemaker. Additionally, the occurrence of alternating bundle-branch block should prompt consideration of a permanent pacemaker. The indications for permanent pacing are unclear, and, like indications for prophylactic temporary pacing, are subject to change as new data become available.

PROTOCOL

Indications for Temporary Pacing

1. Complete heart block with slow ventricular response and wide QRS complex
2. Mobitz type II A-V block with anterior MI
3. Alternating bundle-branch block
4. Right bundle-branch block plus LAFB (new)
5. Right bundle-branch block plus LPFB (new)
6. Recurrent sinus arrest unresponsive to atropine or requiring multiple doses of atropine
7. Sinus bradycardia associated with persistent signs of systemic hypoperfusion and requiring multiple doses of atropine
8. New left bundle-branch block, especially if 1° A-V block is present (controversial)
9. New right bundle-branch block (controversial)

Indications for Permanent Pacing

1. Bifascicular block associated with high-grade A-V block during the course of the infarction
2. Persistent high-grade A-V block after infarction
3. Alternating bundle-branch block during the course of an AMI

Pacemaker catheters may be inserted by way of the right subclavian, external jugular, or femoral veins by the percutaneous Seldinger technique. The position of the lead is probably more stable when these approaches are employed rather than the basilic vein approach.

Recent studies have indicated that the femoral vein route is associated with evidence of venous thrombosis in many instances. The right internal jugular or subclavian routes are currently preferred and appear to be associated with the lowest complication rate. Secure knowledge of the anatomy is a strict requirement of the physician who places the pacemaker in the heart.

PROTOCOL

Insertion of Pacing Catheter
through Right Internal Jugular

1. The patient or next of kin should be informed of the procedure and a note written in the chart explaining the indications and documenting informed consent.

2. The patient is placed supine with the head down. An intravenous line is made secure and running, and the patient is placed on a special fluoroscopy table. The fluoroscopy image intensifier tube is turned on, centered over the heart, and tested for adequate imaging before the procedure begins.

3. The right internal jugular area is prepared with an antiseptic solution, and the patient is draped with sterile towels.

4. Using sterile technique, the operator infiltrates intradermally with 1% lidocaine using a 26-gauge needle. A small incision is made with a No. 11 sharp-pointed scalpel to allow subsequent easy passage of the dilator. A No. 14 needle is then used to infiltrate local anesthetic in the region of the internal jugular vein. Since it is difficult to assess the depth of the vein, small amounts of local anesthetic (about 0.2 mg at a time) should be injected while the needle is advanced slowly.

5. The needle, guide wire, connectors, stylets, syringes, and the like should be tested to ensure that they are all patent. It is particularly important that the pacemaker pass easily through the thin-walled sheath.

6. A sterile 10-ml syringe is connected to the Seldinger needle after the stylet has been removed. When the area has been anesthetized and the equipment is ready, the operator should advance the needle through the previously formed skin incision.

7. Suction is then applied to the syringe, and the needle and syringe are advanced very slowly. A successful puncture is heralded by the appearance of dark venous blood in the syringe.

8. At this point the syringe is disconnected, and the soft tip of the guide wire is inserted through the lumen of the needle provided there is still free flow of blood from the needle. The guide wire should pass easily through the needle and into the internal jugular vein. If it does not, the wire should *not* be forced, because the tip of the needle may be extra-luminal.

9. Once the wire is securely in the vein, the needle is removed and the wire remains. A firm dilator is then passed over the wire, making sure that the firm tip of the guide wire is held beyond the blunt end of the dilator.

10. The dilator is then firmly introduced into the vein over the wire, preparing a pathway for the insertion of the sheath and pacing catheter.

11. When the dilator has been passed through the skin and into the vein, the thin-walled sheath is inserted with the dilator in a firm rotating fashion. The dilator and wire are then removed, and dark venous blood should flow easily from the sheath.

12. The pacing catheter is inserted through the sheath into the internal jugular vein and superior vena cava, where it is visualized by fluoroscopy. The sheath may then be removed from the vein and the catheter advanced to the right atrium.

13. Under fluoroscopic control, a loop is formed in the right atrium, and the catheter is manipulated across the tricuspid valve and into the apex of the right ventricle.

14. The catheter is connected to the external pacing generator. The pacemaker is turned on and the *threshold,* or the smallest amount of milliamperes (mA) necessary to capture the ventricle consistently, is determined. The internal jugular area is then dressed and the catheter secured with adhesive tape or sutures to the skin.

15. Ideally, the initial threshold should allow consistent capture at an energy setting of less than 1 mA. The output should then be set at about twice the threshold. If more than 5 to 6 mA is required for consistent capture, further positioning of the lead should be attempted. Such high milliamperage may be dangerous and can cause ventricular fibrillation in an ischemic myocardium. The sensing threshold should also be assessed using the temporary pulse generator. A two-to threefold margin of safety should be set (i.e., if the endocardial signal measures 10 mV, the setting should be at 3 to 4 mV). The pacemaker should be set on the

demand mode at a rate sufficient to overdrive ectopic foci, usually about 70 to 80 beats per minute

16. Immediately after catheter insertion, a complete 12-lead ECG should be recorded and a chest radiograph obtained. The threshold required to pace should be checked daily by the physician by turning the mA down to the point of noncapture. This threshold value is recorded in the patient's chart. The mA is kept at twice this level. It is not uncommon for the threshold to increase slightly over the first 24 to 48 hours after the pacemaker is inserted.

17. Dressings should be changed and the insertion site examined daily. Some authorities advocate the use of bactericidal ointment on the insertion site.

BIBLIOGRAPHY

Barold, S.S. American College of Cardiology/American Heart Association guidelines for pacemaker implantation after acute myocardial infarction: What is persistent advanced block at the atrioventricular node? *Am. J. Cardiol.* 80:770–774, 1997.

Cheitlin, M.D., Conill, A., Epstein, A.E., et al. ACC/AHA guidelines for implantation of cardiac pacemakers and antiarrhythmia devices. *J. Am. Coll. Cardiol.* 31:1175–1209, 1998.

Ryan, T.J., Anderson, J.L., Antman, E.M., et al. ACC/AHA guidelines for the management of patients with acute myocardial infarction. *J. Am. Coll. Cardiol.* 28:1328–1420, 1996.

Zoll, P.M., Zoll, R.H., Falk, R.H., Clinton, J.E., Eitel, D.R., and Antman, E.M. External noninvasive temporary cardiac pacing: Clinical trials. *Circulation* 71:937–942, 1985.

19

Treatment of Left Ventricular Failure Complicating Myocardial Infarction

The first measurable change during acute myocardial ischemia occurs in *diastole* and is expressed as abnormal left ventricular relaxation. The left ventricular chamber becomes stiffer, and the pressure/volume relationship in the left ventricle is shifted upward and to the left. For any given chamber volume, there is a substantially higher left ventricular end–diastolic pressure (LVEDP) during ischemia or during occlusion of a major coronary artery with an angioplasty balloon catheter. The LVEDP rises abruptly over seconds to minutes.

Much of the "heart failure" that occurs early in the setting of acute myocardial infarction (AMI) is pulmonary congestion on the basis of acute diastolic dysfunction. Often such patients have associated systemic hypertension; they are diaphoretic and tachycardic. The treatment is to quickly reduce pulmonary vascular congestion with a loop diuretic and/or nitroglycerin and to reduce myocardial ischemia with thrombolysis or angioplasty. Blood pressure should be controlled with intravenous nitroglycerin or, in some severe cases, intravenous nitroprusside. The hallmark of diastolic heart failure, which is common in acute ischemic syndromes including AMI, is normal or near normal global LV systolic function by echocardiography and no significant mitral regurgitation. Severe pulmonary edema can occur from diastolic dysfunction, requiring intubation and assisted ventilation.

A second form of heart failure occurs that is even more ominous and is due to severely impaired *systolic* function. This can be transient (stunned myocardium) or permanent (due to severe, extensive myocardial necrosis). Generally but not always, such patients are modestly hypotensive, tachycardic, and relatively oliguric. Like patients with pure diastolic dysfunction, patients with advanced systolic impairment develop pulmonary vascular congestion, tachypnea, and oxygen desaturation. Often these are patients with large anterior MI and substantial wall motion abnormalities by echocardiography.

113

Diastolic heart failure and systolic heart failure can often co-exist. An echocardiogram and the electrocardiogram (ECG) are helpful in differentiating various pathophysiologic substrates such as diastolic heart failure, severe systolic impairment, mitral regurgitation, and right ventricular infarction. In some cases there is a rapid transition from severe systolic impairment to cardiogenic shock. Patients with an AMI and heart failure clearly require close monitoring and often benefit from invasive hemodynamic monitoring including a Swan-Ganz catheter, a Foley catheter to monitor urinary output, and an arterial catheter to monitor blood pressure and blood gases. If there is pulmonary vascular congestion or pulmonary edema, intravenous loop diuretics are indicated. When blood pressure is marginal or even low, intravenous nitroglycerin cannot be employed. Hypotension and impending cardiogenic shock are usually indications for urgent cardiac catheterization. Unless contraindicated, it is prudent to consider patients with systolic heart failure [e.g., cardiac index < 2.5 L/min/m^2 and pulmonary capillary wedge pressure (PCWP) > 15 to 18 mm Hg] for intra-aortic balloon pump (IABP). The counterpulsation technique tends to augment mean arterial pressure, improves coronary blood flow, and reduces left ventricular afterload.

The temptation to employ inotropic therapy for patients with AMI and heart failure should be avoided. The use of such an agent should serve only as a temporary measure prior to placement of an IABP. If such placement is not possible, consideration should be given to transfer of the patient to a center where IABP, urgent catheterization, and surgery are possible. Pressor agents such as high-dose dopamine may temporarily be necessary to help restore blood pressure. However, intra-aortic balloon counterpulsation is the preferred method of stabilizing hemodynamics, not the use of dopamine, dobutamine, or milrinone infusions. Positive inotropic agents tend to increase heart rate and myocardial oxygen demand—unwanted features that are entirely opposite to those of IABP. The goal, of course, is to reduce heart rate and reduce myocardial oxygen demand. There is probably no more powerful tool than IABP in achieving this goal. IABP improves coronary blood flow, blood pressure, cardiac output, renal function, and urine output. Once blood pressure and adequate systemic perfusion is restored with IABP, intravenous nitroglycerin can be cautiously introduced. Urgent cardiac catheterization and coronary angiography should always be considered. Opening up the occluded cul-

prit artery as soon as possible usually helps to further stabilize the patient and improves the prognosis in those with
impending or flank cardiogenic shock (see Chapter 21).

Unless there is extreme systemic hypertension, there is no
role for nitroprusside in the first 48 hours of AMI. It may
divert coronary blood flow away from the region of the
infarct and ischemic regions of the heart, thereby exacer-
bating myocardial ischemia. On the contrary, intravenous
nitroglycerin tends to improve coronary blood flow. The role
of dopamine is primarily to restore blood pressure in a
hypotensive patient prior to insertion of an IABP. Dobutamine and milrinone are reserved for patients with severe
chronic heart failure that has acutely decompensated outside the setting of acute myocardial ischemia or AMI. However, they are sometimes added to help support the failing
circulation in patients with AMI prior to placement of an
IABP and coronary reperfusion in the cath lab.

PROTOCOL
1. A careful physical examination should be performed.
   The chest x-ray and echocardiogram are helpful in determining whether heart failure is due primarily to diastolic dysfunction with pulmonary vascular congestion,
   or whether there is overt or impending severe left ventricular systolic dysfunction and/or mitral regurgitation
   or RV infarct. It is good to remember that systolic and
   diastolic left ventricular dysfunction frequently co-exist.
2. If pulmonary rales are present, intravenous furosemide
   20 to 40 mg should be given. Tachypnea and hypoxemia
   are other indicators of lung congestion and should be
   treated with intravenous furosemide if heart failure is
   suspected. If blood pressure is adequate or elevated,
   intravenous nitroglycerin should be given.
3. When there is evidence of substantially impaired *systolic* function by echocardiography with marginal or low
   blood pressure and pulmonary vascular congestion, the
   patient should be considered for IABP. Some of the LV
   impairment may be due to "myocardial stunning" and
   will either spontaneously improve over days or may
   improve with coronary reperfusion. If frank hypotension
   ensues, intravenous dopamine 5 to 20 µg/kg/min should
   be used to restore blood pressure as quickly as possible
   prior to insertion of an IABP. Intravenous furosemide
   may be necessary to control pulmonary vascular congestion. Dobutamine and milrinone should sometimes
   be considered prior to placement of an IABP and to coro-

nary reperfusion in the cath lab. Nitroprusside is reserved for patients with persistent pump dysfunction beyond the first 48 hours following AMI or is used for those patients with severe hypertension and acute pulmonary edema. Patients with evidence of severely impaired global LV function should be considered for early invasive monitoring with a Swan-Ganz catheter, a Foley catheter, and an arterial line. Urgent or early cardiac catheterization with coronary arteriography and coronary reperfusion are usually indicated following placement of an IABP.

BIBLIOGRAPHY

Boden, W.E., Brooks, W.W., Conrad, C.H., Bing, O.H.L., and Hood, W.B. Jr. Incomplete, delayed functional recovery late after reperfusion following acute myocardial infarction: "Maimed myocardium." *Am. Heart J.* 130:932–933, 1995.

Cohn, J.N. Structural basis for heart failure: ventricular remodeling and its pharmacological inhibition. *Circulation* 91:2504–2507, 1995.

Deedwania, P.C. Prevention of heart failure and post-infarction remodeling. *Congest. Heart Failure* 12:155–164, 1994.

Francis, G.S., and Chu, C. Post-infarction myocardial remodeling: Why does it happen? *Eur. Heart J.* 16 (suppl. N): 31–36, 1995.

Gacioch, G.M., Ellis, S.G., Lee, L., Bates, E.R., Kirsh, M., Walton, J.A., and Topol, E.J. Cardiogenic shock complicating acute myocardial infarction: The use of coronary angioplasty and the integration of the new support devices into patient management. *J. Am. Coll. Cardiol.* 19: 647–653, 1992.

Gaudron, P., Eilles, C., Ertl, G., and Kochsiek, K. Compensatory and noncompensatory left ventricular dilatation after myocardial infarction: Time course and hemodynamic consequences at rest and during exercise. *Am. Heart J.* 123:337–385, 1992.

Gaudron, P., Eilles, C., Kugler, I., and Ertl, G. Progressive left ventricular dysfunction and remodeling after myocardial infarction: Potential mechanisms and early predictors. *Circulation* 87:755–763, 1993.

Genton, R., and Jaffee, A.S. Management of congestive heart failure in patients with acute myocardial infarction. *J. A. M. A.* 256:2556–2560, 1986.

Kloner, R.A., Bolli, R., Marban, E., Reinlib, L., and Braunwald, E. Medical and cellular implications of stunning, hibernation and preconditioning. *Circulation* 97: 1848–1867, 1998.

Lee, L.K., Woodlief, L.H., Topol, E.J., et al. Predictors of 30-day mortality in the era of reperfusion for acute myocardial infarction: Results from an international trial of 41,021 patients. *Circulation* 91:1659–1668, 1995.

McKay, R.G., Pfeffer, M.A., Pasternak, R.C., et al. Left ventricular remodeling after myocardial infarction: A corollary to infarct expansion. *Circulation* 74:693–702, 1986.

Nakamura, S., Iwasaka, T., Sugiura, T., Ohkubo, N., Tsuji, H., and Inada, M. Natural history of left ventricular function in patients with uncomplicated acute myocardial infarction. *Chest* 103:1320–1324, 1993.

O'Connor, C.M., Hathaway, W.R., Bates, E., et al. Clinical characteristics and long-term outcome of patients in whom congestive heart failure develops after thrombolytic therapy for acute myocardial infarction: Development of a predictive model. *Am. Heart J.* 133:663–673, 1997.

Pfeffer, M.A., and Braunwald, E. Ventricular enlargement following infarction is a modifiable Process. *Am. J. Cardiol.* 68:127D–131D, 1991.

Pfeffer, M.A., and Braunwald, E. Ventricular remodeling after myocardial infarction: Experimental observations and clinical implications. *Circulation* 81:1161–1172, 1990.

Popovic, A.D., Neŝkovic, A. N., Marinkovic, J., Lee, J.C., Tan, M., and Thomas, J.D. Serial assessment of left ventricular chamber stiffness after acute myocardial infarction. *Am. J. Cardiol.* 77:361–364, 1996.

Warren, S.E., Royal, H.D., Markis, J.E., Grossman, W., and McKay, R.G. Time course of left ventricular dilation after myocardial infarction: Influence of infarct-related artery and success of coronary thrombolysis. *J. Am. Coll. Cardiol.* 11:12–19, 1988.

Weisman, H.F., Bush, D.E., Mannisi, J.A., Weisfeldt, M.L., and Healy, B. Cellular mechanisms of myocardial infarct expansion. *Circulation* 78:186–201, 1988.

20

Treatment of Acute Mitral Regurgitation and Ventricular Septal Rupture

A systolic murmur associated with signs and symptoms of severe left ventricular failure developing in a patient with an acute myocardial infarction (AMI) is highly suggestive of acute mitral regurgitation or rupture of the ventricular septum.

Patients with rupture of an entire papillary muscle deteriorate rapidly despite intensive medical management. Papillary muscle dysfunction or the rupture of only one or two chordae tendineae can be associated with severe left ventricular failure, but the patient's demise is not quite so precipitous as with rupture of an entire papillary muscle. Patients with rupture (tear) of the ventricular septum have a clinical course similar to that seen with papillary muscle dysfunction or subtotal papillary muscle rupture.

It may be difficult to differentiate between the murmurs of acute mitral regurgitation (MR) and ventricular septal rupture. A bedside echo-Doppler examination often reveals the correct diagnosis. Patients with rupture of the ventricular septum invariably have a loud systolic murmur that is often localized or at least maximal in intensity at the lower left sternal border. However, some patients with MR may manifest only a soft systolic murmur. Occasionally, patients with severe MR have no audible systolic murmur. Such patients with severe but silent MR have very poor left ventricular function. Even individuals with silent or barely audible murmurs of mitral regurgitation usually demonstrate large V waves in the tracing of pulmonary capillary wedge pressure (PCWP). Hence, a pulmonary arterial catheter should be inserted in all patients suspected of having sustained one of these two complications. An arterial line is almost always required as well. A Foley catheter is frequently helpful in monitoring urine output in these critically ill patients.

Patients with severe MR or ventricular septal rupture and left ventricular failure require aggressive medical and often surgical therapy. Before embarking on such a course, the physician should ascertain that the patient is an appropriate candidate for such aggressive diagnostic and therapeutic interventions. Factors that militate strongly against an aggressive approach include: poor left ventricular function; profound and prolonged hypotension, particularly if it is accompanied by renal insufficiency or acute tubular necrosis; age greater than 75 years (this is a relative negative factor and can be overridden by an elderly patient's vitality and previous good health); chronic illness, and cachexia. The physician must evaluate each patient carefully and decide whether aggressive management is indicated.

PROTOCOL

1. Obtain an echo-Doppler study at the bedside.
2. Pulmonary arterial and systemic arterial catheters are usually inserted. Serial, duplicate 2-ml blood samples should be obtained in heparinized syringes from the superior vena cava, right atrium, right ventricle, and pulmonary artery as the balloon catheter is advanced. These samples should be free of air bubbles, capped, and preserved on ice until percent oxygen saturation determinations can be made. It is not necessary to discontinue supplemental inspiratory oxygen.
3. The presence of a significant increase (or "step-up") in right ventricular oxygen saturation (as compared with right atrial values) is diagnostic of ventricular septal rupture. The absence of a step-up combined with the presence of large V waves in the PCWP tracing implies significant acute MR. The echo-Doppler study can also help to quantitate shunt or regurgitant blood flow. Patients with ventricular septal defect (VSD) and a large left-to-right shunt frequently have large V waves in the PCWP tracing. Thus, the presence or absence of a step-up in right ventricular hemoglobin oxygen saturation is the crucial finding for making the diagnosis of VSD by right heart catheterization.
4. To determine whether a patient has a significant oxygen step-up, blood samples are obtained from the superior vena cava, right atrium, right ventricle, and pulmonary artery, as described in paragraph 2, above. The oxygen content of all samples is calculated as follows: oxygen content of the sample in volumes per milliliter = hemoglobin (g/ml) × 1.39 × percent saturation of the sample. A difference of greater than 1 vol/ml between the right atrium and the right ventricle signifies a significant left-to-right shunt from a ventricular septal rupture. The amount of blood shunting left to right can be calculated from the following formulas:

    a. Left-to-right shunt = (pulmonary blood flow) – (systemic blood flow)

    b. Pulmonary blood flow = oxygen consumption ÷ (arterial blood oxygen content) – (pulmonary arterial blood oxygen content)

    c. Systemic blood flow = oxygen consumption ÷ (arterial blood oxygen content)–(right atrial blood oxygen content). Oxygen consumption is determined with a Douglas bag and the help of the catheterization laboratory, or an assumed value may be obtained from Appendix III. The patient's body surface area in meters squared can easily be determined from a nomogram if one knows the person's height and weight (see Appendix II).

5. The treatment for acute MR and ventricular septal rupture is similar. It consists of attempts to "compensate" the left ventricle and allow for elective surgical correction at a later date (usually 3 months if compensation can be achieved).

    a. Milder forms of MR and ventricular septal rupture produce left ventricular failure, which can often be controlled temporarily with vasodilators, digitalis, and diuretics. Vasodilator agents such as angiotensin-converting enzyme inhibitors, or occasionally isosorbide dinitrate and hydralazine in combination, together with diuretics constitute the most important components of pharmacologic therapy.

    b. More severe forms of MR and ventricular septal rupture are associated with considerable degrees of left ventricular failure (PCWP of > 20 mm Hg, cardiac index < 2.0 L/min/m²), requiring more aggressive management.

6. A nitroprusside infusion should be initiated (intraarterial pressure monitoring is essential) at 15 µg/min and the drip rate increased at intervals of 3 to 5 minutes until the PCWP falls below 18 mm Hg. Systolic arterial pressure should not fall below 90 to 95 mm Hg. It is rarely necessary to infuse more than 200 µg/min of nitroprusside.

7. Most authorities feel that nitroprusside is contraindicated in hypotensive patients. Dopamine, dobutamine, or amrinone infusion should be instituted as described in the protocol for cardiogenic shock (see Chapter 21). Some authorities have employed a combination of

dopamine or dobutamine and nitroprusside in these patients.

8. Intra-aortic balloon counterpulsation is strongly recommended unless contraindicated (e.g., severe obliterative peripheral vascular disease). The catheterization laboratory and the cardiac surgical team should be consulted.

9. Cardiac surgical repair (mitral valve replacement or closure of ventricular septal rupture) is usually performed as soon as possible. However, selected patients who are very stable without tachycardia or clinical signs of congestive heart failure can be monitored closely until they are over the acute phase of the MI (3 to 6 weeks). Surgery is performed at that time. However, most of these patients require urgent catheterization and surgery. Coronary artery bypass grafting is usually performed along with the repair procedure (see Chapter 30).

10. Patients with severe heart failure or shock should undergo surgery as rapidly as possible.

BIBLIOGRAPHY

Braunwald, E. Mitral regurgitation: Physiologic, clinical and surgical considerations. *N. Engl. J. Med.* 281: 425–433, 1969.

Burch, G.E., DePasquale, N.P., and Phillips, J.H. The syndrome of papillary muscle dysfunction. *Am. Heart J.* 75: 399–415, 1968.

Calvo, F.E., Figueras, J., Cortadellas, J., and Soler-Soler, J. Severe mitral regurgitation complicating acute myocardial infarction: Clinical and angiographic differences between patients with and without papillary muscle rupture. *Eur. Heart J.* 18:1606–1610, 1997.

Figueras, J., Cortadellas, J., Calvo, F., and Soler-Soler, J. Relevance of delayed hospital admission on development of cardiac rupture during acute myocardial infarction: Study in 225 patients with free wall, septal or papillary muscle rupture. *J. Am. Coll. Cardiol.* 32:135–139, 1998.

Goldman, M.E., Horowitz, S.F., Meller, J., Mindich, B., and Teichholz, L.E. Recovery of right ventricular function following repair of acute ventricular septal defect. *Chest* 82:59–63, 1982.

Held, A.C., Cole, P.L., Lipton, B., et al. Rupture of the interventricular septum complicating acute myocardial infarction: A multicenter analysis of clinical findings and outcome. *Am. Heart J.* 116:1330–1336, 1988.

Hendren, W.G., Nemec, J.J., Lytle, B.W., et al. Mitral valve repair for ischemic mitral insufficiency. *Ann. Thorac. Surg.* 52:1246–1251, 1991.

Kishon, Y., Oh, J.K., Schaff, H.V., Mullany, C.J., Tajik, A.J., and Gersh, B.J. Mitral valve operation in post-infarction rupture of a papillary muscle: Immediate results and long-term follow-up of 22 patients. *Mayo Clin. Proc.* 67: 1023–1030, 1992.

Lamas, G.A., Mitchell, G.F., Flaker, G.C., Smith, S.C. Jr., Gersh, B.J., Basta, L., et al. Clinical significance of mitral regurgitation after acute myocardial infarction. *Circulation* 96:827–833, 1997.

Lehmann, K.G., Francis, C.K., Dodge, H.T., and the TIMI Study Group. Mitral regurgitation in early myocardial infarction—Incidence, clinical detection, and prognostic implications. *Ann. Intern. Med.* 117: 10–17, 1992.

Lemery, R., Smith, H.C., Giuliani, E.R., and Gersh, B.J. Prognosis in rupture of the ventricular septum after acute myocardial infarction and role of early surgical intervention. *Am. J. Cardiol.* 70:147–151, 1992.

Montoya, A., McKeever, L., Scanlon, P., Sullivan, H.J., Gunnar, R.M., and Roque, P. Early repair of ventricular septal rupture after infarction. *Am. J. Cardiol.* 45:345–348, 1980.

Nishimura, R.A., Schaff, H.V., Shub, C., Gersh, B.J., Edwards, W.D., and Tajik, A.J. Papillary muscle rupture complicating acute myocardial infarction: Analysis of 17 patients. *Am. J. Cardiol.* 51:373–377, 1983.

Skillington, P.D., Davies, R.H., Luff, A.J., et al. Surgical treatment for infarct-related ventricular septal defects: Improved early results combined with analysis of late functional status. *J. Thorac. Cardiovasc. Surg.* 99:798–808, 1990.

Tcheng, J.E., Jackman, J.J., Nelson, C.L., et al. Outcome of patients sustaining acute ischemic mitral regurgitation during myocardial infarction. *Ann. Intern. Med.* 117: 18–24, 1992.

Wei, J.Y., Hutchins, G.M., and Bulkley, B.H. Papillary muscle rupture in fatal acute myocardial infarction—A potentially treatable form of cardiogenic shock. *Ann. Intern. Med.* 90:149–153, 1979.

Westaby, S., Parry, A., Ormerod, O., Gooneratne, P., and Pillai, R. Thrombolysis and postinfarction ventricular septal rupture. *J. Thorac. Cardiovasc. Surg.* 104:1506–1509, 1992.

21

Treatment of Suspected Cardiogenic Shock

Cardiogenic shock (CGS) is the most dreaded complication of acute myocardial infarction (AMI), with a mortality frequently in excess of 90%. This entity occurs when approximately 40% of the left ventricular myocardium is rendered nonfunctional by necrosis and ischemia. Recent data indicate that the prognosis of cardiogenic shock can be substantially improved by opening up the "culprit" artery with percutaneous transluminal coronary angioplasty (PTCA). Once the diagnosis of cardiogenic shock is suspected, the patient should be promptly referred for PTCA. Blood pressure should be stabilized with dopamine, if possible, before attempting PTCA. Uncontrolled studies indicate that this aggressive strategy can lower mortality from 80% to 90% to 30% to 50%.

The clinical criteria defining CGS are clearly important if accurate assessment of various forms of therapy is to be achieved. The incidence of CGS and the results of therapy vary in different clinical centers because of differences in the definition of CGS. The following criteria for CGS reflect current established definitions of this entity:

1. The diagnosis of MI by the usual clinical data [i.e., history, physical examination, electrocardiogram (ECG)].
2. Systolic blood pressure less than 90 mm Hg by cuff on two successive determinations. However, a higher pressure (e.g., 100 mm Hg) may occur in previously hypertensive patients.
3. Urine output less than 20 to 30 ml/h.
4. Absence of other causes of hypotension such as:
   a. Overenthusiastic dosage of quinidine, procainamide, diuretics, or antihypertensive medications
   b. Arrhythmias
   c. Significant disorders of electrolytes, acid-base balance, and arterial blood gases
   d. Dehydration or bradycardia-hypotension syndrome (see "Protocol" below, item 1).
5. Presence of clinical signs of shock, such as depressed mentation and peripheral vasoconstriction (e.g., pallid or mottled, cool, clammy skin).

Therapeutic efforts for patients with cardiogenic shock have often been discouragingly ineffective. Temporary improvement in the patient's condition can be obtained with intra-aortic balloon counterpulsation, although subsequent deterioration and death are generally the rule. Recently, a number of uncontrolled reports have suggested that mechanical or pharmacologic thrombolysis combined with intra-aortic counterpulsation can improve the prognosis for patients with cardiogenic shock secondary to MI. Such therapy should be initiated within 4 hours of the onset of shock in order to be effective. It is exceedingly unlikely that thrombolysis will benefit a patient who has been in cardiogenic shock for many hours, particularly if incipient renal insufficiency is present.

PROTOCOL

1. All patients with suspected CGS should have a pulmonary arterial catheter placed by way of the neck, arm, or leg (see Chapter 26). The pulmonary capillary wedge pressure (PCWP) (confirmed by a similar pulmonary arterial diastolic pressure unless the patient has significant chronic obstructive pulmonary disease) should be 15 to 18 mm Hg or more. Patients with values less than this are either dehydrated (e.g., from chronic diuretic use) or have the bradycardia-hypotension syndrome (Bezold-Jarisch reflex, which is particularly common with inferior MIs). The latter two groups of patients should be infused with either crystalloid (NaCl solution), albumin, plasma, or low molecular-weight dextran until a PCWP of approximately 18 mm Hg is obtained. Dextrose in water and saline can leak across capillary membranes and hence may be only transient in effectiveness. Significant bradycardia should be treated with intravenous atropine or pacing (see Chapters 12 and 13).

2. In all patients with suspected CGS, an arterial line should be placed, with the lumen as close to the aorta as possible. Peripheral arterial pressures (e.g., radial artery) can be misleading. Relatively long catheters inserted from the radial, brachial, or femoral arteries are preferred. Slow, continuous low-dose heparin infusion (1 U/ml in 5% D/W or saline) should be instituted through both systemic arterial and pulmonary arterial catheters. A Foley catheter should also be inserted to aid in monitoring urine output.

3. While systemic arterial and pulmonary arterial lines are being introduced into the patient in order to assess the severity of the shock state and the left ventricular filling pressure, it is frequently prudent to support the systemic blood pressure pharmacologically with dopamine, dobutamine, norepinephrine, amrinone, or various combinations of these agents (e.g., dopamine plus dobutamine) (see item 4a, below). If the patient is subsequently found (by pulmonary arterial catheterization) to be hypovolemic, these pressor agents can gradually be tapered while appropriate volume therapy is administered.

4. The treatment of patients in whom intra-arterial pressures and clinical data support the diagnosis of CGS is as follows:

   a. A trial of dopamine or dobutamine infusion is instituted, starting with 3 to 5 µg/kg/min (or 3 to 10 µg/kg/min of dobutamine) and increasing the dose to 20 to 50 µg/kg/min (20 to 40 µg/kg/min of dobutamine) if an inadequate response is obtained. If the response is still inadequate, a trial infusion of both agents simultaneously or of norepinephrine (Levophed), 2 to 8 µg/min, is warranted. (Note that the total dosage is 2 to 8 µg/min, *not* 2 to 8 µg/kg/min.) Isoproterenol is contraindicated (see Chapter 12). Patients with milder degrees of hypotension (80 to 90 mm Hg) may respond to dobutamine; more profound degrees of hypotension require therapy with dopamine or Levophed.

   b. Patients should be promptly brought to the cardiac catheterization lab. Attempts to open the occluded artery with PTCA should be performed.

   c. Intra-aortic balloon counterpulsation should be strongly considered. Cardiac surgery should be consulted if appropriate.

5. The benefit of digitalis, diuretics, and anticoagulants in CGS patients is marginal at best.

6. Patients with CGS frequently benefit from intra-aortic balloon counterpulsation. Some patients in CGS are candidates for emergency coronary artery bypass grafts. Patients with left main or severe three-vessel coronary artery disease, individuals in whom the CGS state is severe, or those who fail to improve rapidly after initiation of counterpulsation and PTCA should be considered for coronary artery bypass grafting. Patients with mechanical complications of AMI (i.e., mitral regurgita-

tion or ventricular septal rupture) associated with CGS frequently benefit from surgical intervention. Patients with diffuse left ventricular hypokinesis and akinesis and no mechanical complication of AMI are usually not candidates for surgical intervention but may benefit from PTCA.

a. Patients should be transferred to the catheterization laboratory, and the procedure should be performed during intra-aortic counterpulsation. The patient may either be returned to the CCU following the catheterization or sent directly to the operating room (see Chapter 30). If catheterization is performed, it should be undertaken as soon as possible after the development of CGS.

BIBLIOGRAPHY

Allen, B.S., Buckberg, G.D., Fontan, F.M., et al. Superiority of controlled surgical reperfusion versus percutaneous transluminal coronary angioplasty in acute coronary occlusion. *J. Thorac. Cardiovasc. Surg.* 105:864–884, 1993.

Alonso, D.R., Scheidt, S., Post, M., and Killip, T. Pathophysiology of cardiogenic shock: Quantification of myocardial necrosis, clinical, pathologic and electrocardiographic correlations. *Circulation* 48:588–596, 1973.

Barry, W.L., and Sarembock, I.J. Cardiogenic shock: Therapy and prevention. *Clin. Cardiol.* 21:72–80, 1998.

Bates, E.R., and Topol, E.J. Limitations of thrombolytic therapy for acute myocardial infarction complicated by congestive heart failure and cardiogenic shock. *J. Am. Coll. Cardiol.* 18:1077–1084, 1991.

Bengston, J.R., Kaplan, A.J., Pieper, K.S., et al. Prognosis in cardiogenic shock after acute myocardial infarction in the interventional era. *J. Am. Coll. Cardiol.* 20:1482–1489, 1992.

Berger, P.B., Holmes, D.R., Stebbins, A.L., et al. Impact of an aggressive invasive catheterization and revascularization strategy on mortality in patients with cardiogenic shock in the GUSTO-I trial. *Circulation* 96:122–127, 1997.

Berger, P.B., Tuttle, R.H., Holmes, D.R. Jr., et al. One year survival among patients with acute myocardial infarction complicated by cardiogenic shock, and its relation to early revascularization: Results from the GUSTO-I trial. *Circulation* 99:873–878, 1999.

Gacioch, G.M., Ellis, S.G., Lee, L., et al. Cardiogenic shock complicating acute myocardial infarction: The use of coronary angioplasty and the integration of the new support devices into patient management. *J. Am. Coll. Cardiol.* 19:647–653, 1992.

Goldberg, R.J., Gore, J.M., Alpert, J.S., et al. Cardiogenic shock after acute myocardial infarction. *N. Engl. J. Med.* 325:1117–1122, 1991.

Hands, M.E., Rutherford, J.D., Muller, J.E., et al., and the Milis Study Group. The in-hospital development of cardiogenic shock after myocardial infarction: Incidence, predictors of occurrence, outcome and prognostic factors. *J. Am. Coll. Cardiol.* 14:40–46, 1989.

Hasdal, D., Holmes, D.R. Jr., Topol, E.J., et al. Frequency and clinical outcome of cardiogenic shock during acute myocardial infarction among patients receiving reteplase or alteplase: Results from GUSTO-III. *Eur. Heart J.* 20:128–135, 1999.

Hibbard, M.D., Holmes, D.R., Bailey, K.R., Reeder, G.S., Bresnahan, J.F., and Gersh, B.J. Percutaneous transluminal coronary angioplasty in patients with cardiogenic shock. *J. Am. Coll. Cardiol.* 19:639–646, 1992.

Hochman, J.S., Boland, J., Sleeper, L.A., et al. Current spectrum of cardiogenic shock and effect of early revascularization on mortality: Results of an International Registry. SHOCK Registry Investigators. *Circulation* 91:873–881, 1995.

Klein, L.W. Optimal therapy for cardiogenic shock: The emerging role of coronary angioplasty (editorial). *J. Am. Coll. Cardiol.* 19:654–656, 1992.

Kovack, P.J., Rasak, M.A., Bates, E.R., Ohman, E.M., and Stomel, R.J. Thrombolysis plus aortic counterpulsation: Improved survival in patients who present to community hospital with cardiogenic shock. *J. Am. Coll. Cardiol.* 29:1454–1458, 1997.

Lee, L., Erbel, R., Brown, T.M., Laufer, N., Meyer, J., and O'Neill, W.W. Multicenter registry of angioplasty therapy of cardiogenic shock: Initial and long-term survival. *J. Am. Coll. Cardiol.* 17:599–603, 1991.

Page, D.L., Caulfield, J.J., Kastor, J.A., DeSanctis, R.W., and Saunders, C.A. Myocardial changes associated with cardiogenic shock. *N. Engl. J. Med.* 285:133–137, 1971.

22

Treatment of Hypertension Complicating Acute Myocardial Infarction

It is well known that arterial blood pressure (BP) is an important determinant of myocardial oxygen demand. Therefore there has been a long-standing belief that control of high blood pressure in the setting of acute myocardial infarction (AMI) is quite important. Patients are frequently admitted to the emergency department and the coronary care unit (CCU) with a combination of severe hypertension and AMI. In GUSTO, the incidence of total stroke and intracranial hemorrhage was related to systolic BP at entry. When systolic BP was 175 mm Hg or more, the incidence of total stroke rose from 1.17% to 3.4%. Of course, severe hypertension also precludes the use of thrombolytic therapy. It is unknown whether reduction of very high BP pressure with intravenous vasodilators allows for the safe delivery of thrombolytic therapy. Usually BP gradually diminishes with the use of morphine sulfate to control pain. Moreover, the use of intravenous nitroglycerin and intravenous beta-adrenergic blockers adds further to the diminishment of BP. By the time the patient is admitted to the CCU, BP is usually under reasonable control.

Persistence of high BP (>140/90) is usually due to inadequately treated severe discomfort and anxiety. The approach to this problem is usually to add more analgesics. Pain that is not easily relieved might be due to other conditions, such as acute aortic dissection, which should always be considered and excluded. Acute pulmonary edema is often accompanied by severe hypertension. For those patients who demonstrate high BP despite the control of pain and anxiety, additional anti-hypertensive therapy is usually necessary. Nitroprusside might be considered, but it is possible that this vasodilator may aggravate acute myocardial ischemia by redirecting coronary blood flow away from the ischemic segment and toward the more normally perfused part of the heart. High doses of intravenous nitroglycerin in conjunction with intravenous beta-adrenergic blockers may be more appropriate for severe hypertension accompanying AMI. Re-institution of oral anti-hypertensive drugs may be necessary in patients with an antecedent history of high BP.

Angiotensin-converting enzyme (ACE) inhibitors, which are now commonly used in the post-infarction setting, may be employed straight away. Enalaprilat can be given intravenously, but oral ACE inhibitor therapy is usually sufficient. The liberal use of intravenous beta-adrenergic blockers should be strongly considered in such patients unless there are contraindications to their use.

PROTOCOL

1. Patients with AMI whose BPs are in excess of 140/90 mm Hg on admission to the CCU should be treated as follows:
   a. Sufficient sedation and analgesia should be provided to completely relieve anxiety and chest discomfort. This is usually in the form of morphine sulfate.
   b. Sublingual and intravenous nitroglycerin can be employed, which will help to alleviate discomfort and lower blood pressure.
   c. The liberal use of beta-adrenergic blockers should be considered unless contraindicated. These can be given intravenously if necessary, with subsequent use of oral agents once BP has been controlled.
2. Patients with extreme hypertension who are at risk for cerebrovascular events or myocardial rupture should be considered for treatment with intravenous nitroprusside. However, nitroprusside is rarely indicated in the setting AMI; moreover, it can aggravate myocardial ischemia due to diversion of blood away from ischemic segments and toward more normal myocardial segments.
3. If high BP cannot be controlled with a combination of analgesia, anxiolytic agents, intravenous nitroglycerin, and intravenous beta blockers, one should consider adding more standard anti-hypertensive agents such as ACE inhibitors. Intravenous enalaprilat can be used, but oral agents are usually sufficient.

BIBLIOGRAPHY

Ayward, P.E., Wilcox, R.G., Horgan, J.H., et al. Relation of increased arterial blood pressure to mortality and stroke in the context of contemporary thrombolytic therapy for acute myocardial infarction: A randomized trial. GUSTO-I Investigators. *Ann. Intern. Med.* 125:891–900, 1996.

Bodenheimer, M.M., Ramanathan, K., Banka, V.S., and Helfant, R.H. Effect of progressive pressure reduction with nitroprusside on acute myocardial infarction in humans: Determination of optimal afterload. *Ann. Intern. Med.* 94:435–439, 1981.

Dunn, F.G. Hypertension and myocardial infarction. *J. Am. Coll. Cardiol.* 1:528–532, 1983.

Hillis, L.D., Izquierdo, C., Davis, C., et al. Effect of various degrees of systemic arterial hypertension on acute canine myocardial ischemia. *Am. J. Physiol.* 240:H855–H861, 1981.

Roan, P.G., Buja, M., Saffer, S., et al. Effects of systemic hypertension on ischemic and nonischemic regional left ventricular function in awake, unsedated dogs after experimental coronary occlusion. *Circulation* 66:115–125, 1982.

Wantanabe, T., Covell, J.W., Maroko, P.R., Braunwald, E., and Ross, J. Jr. Effects of increased arterial pressure and positive inotropic agents on the severity of myocardial ischemia in the acutely depressed heart. *Am. J. Cardiol.* 50:371–377, 1972.

23

Treatment of Unstable Angina

Unstable angina, also referred to as *acute coronary syndrome,* is a common reason for patients to be admitted to the coronary care unit (CCU). The definition of unstable coronary artery syndrome varies substantially. Some cardiologists include non–ST-T-wave elevation MI, while others consider this separate from unstable angina. Patients with unstable angina typically present with chest discomfort, either new or progressive angina associated with transient ST-segment depression on the electrocardiogram (ECG) but without evidence of myocardial infarction by creatine kinase (CK) or CK-MB iso-enzymes. Many patients have a rise in troponin T or I with no abnormality of CK-MB, a marker of a poorer prognosis.

It is important to perform a 12-lead ECG during chest pain. Serum markers of acute myocardial injury should be sequentially measured. In patients with ST-segment elevation, acute reperfusion is imperative. In patients without ST-segment elevation, there is no evidence that urgent coronary reperfusion is beneficial. With the recent use of troponin measurements, the distinction between unstable angina and myocardial infarction has become less clear. Many patients previously categorized as having unstable angina are now known to have small amounts of myocardial necrosis as measured by elevated troponin levels.

The treatment of unstable angina continues to evolve. The basic elements include the use of agents to antagonize platelet aggregation (aspirin or clopidogrel), agents that inhibit thrombin production (still in clinical trials), agents to improve coronary blood flow and reduce wall stress (intravenous nitrates), and beta-adrenergic blockers to reduce myocardial oxygen demand (intravenous metoprolol). Intravenous heparin is widely used to treat unstable angina, although the strength of the evidence for its use is much lower than that for aspirin. Thrombosis can be reactivated when heparin is discontinued, so it should not be stopped unless aspirin is "on board." Low-molecular-weight heparin may be superior or equivalent to unfractionated heparin, and its role for the treatment of unstable angina is still evolving. The most hotly contested issue, however, is that of when to perform revascularization. If pain with ST-T changes persists or is recurrent on maximal therapy, the intra-aortic balloon pump may be helpful. If symptoms persist despite maximal therapy, diagnostic coronary angiography with an eye toward coronary reperfusion may become urgent.

The risk of unstable angina is variable, the event rate of patients over the age of 65 being twice that of patients below age 65 (Table 23-1). About 50% to 60% of patients undergo coronary angiography during hospitalization, with about 20% of patients receiving angioplasty and 15% undergoing surgery.

The occlusive thrombus that characterizes acute coronary syndromes, including myocardial infarction (MI), consists of a platelet-rich core (white clot) and a bulkier surrounding fibrin-rich (red) clot. Plasminogen activators, such as tissue plasminogen activator (t-PA), restore vessel patency by lysing the fibrin-rich red clot, but they do not affect the platelet-rich white clot and are not indicated for the treatment of unstable angina. In fact, fibrinolysis tends to expose thrombus, a potent platelet activator. The glycoprotein IIb/IIIa inhibitors abciximab (ReoPro), tirofiban (Aggrastat) and eptifibatide (Integrilin) have all been studied in large trials and are now used for treatment of patients with acute coronary syndromes.

The monoclonal antibody to the IIb/IIIa receptor abciximab (ReoPro) binds very tightly to the IIb/IIIa and vitronectin receptors, and the anti-platelet effect lasts much longer than the infusion period. If bleeding occurs, stopping the drug does not immediately reverse the anti-platelet effect. Transfusion of platelets redistributes the antibodies among all the platelets, thereby reducing the level of platelet inhibition. The peptide (tirofiban) and peptidomimetic (eptifibatide) agents are competitive inhibitors of the IIb/IIIa receptors, and have much shorter half-lives than axciximab; when the infusion is stopped, the anti-platelet activity reverses in a few hours. Abciximab is widely used in conjunction with angioplasty and stent deployment in the cath lab, whereas tirofiban and eptifibatide are more commonly used for unstable angina without associated cath lab intervention. The role of tirofiban and eptifibatide, short-acting IIb/IIIa antagonists, is still evolving in the treatment of unstable angina (see PRISM, PRISM-Plus, and PURSUIT Trials in the bibliography at the end of this chapter).

Last, it is becoming increasingly clear that patients with acute coronary syndromes including unstable angina, benefit from HMG-CoA reductase inhibitors ("statins"). Benefit is

Table 23-1.   Short-term risk of death or nonfatal myocardial infarction in patients with symptoms suggestive of unstable angina

High risk	Intermediate risk	Low risk
At least one of the following features must be present:	No high-risk feature but any of the following:	No high- or intermediate-risk feature but may have any of the following:
Prolonged ongoing (>20 min) rest pain	Rest angina now resolved but not low likelihood of CAD	Increased angina frequency, severity, or duration
Pulmonary edema	Rest angina (>20 min) or relieved with rest or nitroglycerin	Angina provoked at a lower threshold
Angina with new or worsening mitral regurgitation murmur	Angina with dynamic T wave changes	New-onset angina within 2 weeks to 2 months
Rest angina with dynamic ST-changes ≥1 mm	Nocturnal angina	Normal or unchanged ECG
Angina with S_3 or rales	New onset rest angina or angina with minimal activity but low likelihood of CAD	
Angina with hypotension	Q waves or ST-segment depression ≥1 mm in multiple leads; Age > 65 years	

CAD, coronary artery disease; ECG, electrocardiogram.
(Adapted from *Clinical Practice Guideline: Diagnosing and Managing Unstable Angina, Agency for Health Care Policy and Research.* Publication No. 94-0603. Bethesda, MD: National Heart, Lung, and Blood Institute, 1994.)

derived even by patients with "normal" cholesterol levels. This secondary prevention measure reduces coronary events, strokes, and overall mortality. The statins appear to improve endothelial function and may stabilize coronary plaques through mechanisms unrelated to their cholesterol-lowering properties.

PROTOCOL

1. Patients with unstable angina should be admitted to the CCU if they are at high-risk (Table 23-1) or have angina with ECG changes. A 12-lead ECG should be performed during episodes of angina.

2. Aspirin-naive patients should be given 324 mg of *non-enteric* acetylsalicylic acid (ASA) to chew and swallow as soon as possible, and should be continued on one aspirin per day. Patients already receiving aspirin daily should be continued on at least 80 mg of aspirin per day.

3. Sublingual nitroglycerin should be given if the patient is having angina.

4. Intravenous nitroglycerin should be started at 10 to 20 µg/min and increased by 5 to 10 µg/min every 5 to 10 minutes until angina diminishes. The mean aortic blood pressure should be maintained in the range of 70 to 80 mm Hg if possible.

5. Intravenous metoprolol 5 to 10 mg should be used as needed to reduce heart rate and blood pressure unless contraindicated. The dose varies widely from patient to patient. When stable, patients should be switched to oral beta-adrenergic blockers (i.e., metoprolol 25 to 100 mg b.i.d.).

6. Intravenous heparin (unfractionated) 5000 units should be given by bolus, followed by 1000 units per hour and adjusted after 6, 12, 24, 36, and 48 hours to an activated partial thromboplastin time of 50 to 75 seconds. A weight-adjusted nomogram can also be used, starting with a dose of 80 U/kg followed by an infusion of 18 U/kg/h. For patients weighing less than 70 kg, even lower doses are sometimes recommended (i.e., 60 U/kg bolus followed by 12 U/kg/h). The target therapeutic range is still 50 to 75 seconds. Various low-molecular-weight heparin preparations may be superior to unfractionated heparin in unstable angina. Their use does not usually require monitoring of the aPTT. If catheterization with intervention or cardiac surgery is anticipated, unfractionated heparin may be preferred, as it is readily reversible. If the patient is unlikely to need an inva-

sive procedure (percutaneous coronary intervention) or surgery, one might consider the use of a low-molecular-weight heparin such as enoxiparin 1 mg/kg subcutaneously b.i.d. for 2 to 8 days.

7. Use of an intra-aortic balloon pump may be necessary for patients who fail to respond to conventional medical therapy.

8. IIb/IIIa platelet antagonists are emerging as an important new therapy for unstable angina. Abciximab (Reo Pro), which is long-acting, is primarily being used in conjunction with cath lab–based interventional procedures. Tirofiban (Aggrastat) and eptifibatide (Integrilin) are short-acting IIb/IIIa antagonists and are used for unstable angina, with or without intervention. The IIb/IIIa antagonists are sensitive to renal insufficiency, and their dose should be adjusted accordingly. These agents can occasionally cause severe thrombocytopenia and have a number of clear contra-indications that are roughly similar to those for thrombolytic therapy but also include renal failure.

   Abciximab (Reo Pro) is given as a 0.25-mg/kg bolus followed by 0.125 µg/kg/min infusion for 12 hours; it is used with heparin 100 U/kg bolus plus additional heparin to achieve a procedural activated coagulation time (ACT) of at least 300 seconds, or sometimes with low-dose heparin 70 units/kg with additional heparin to achieve an ACT target of at least 200 seconds. Eptifibatide (Integrilin) is given as a 180 µg/kg bolus followed by a 2 µg/kg/min infusion for 72 hours. A smaller dose of 135 µg/kg bolus and 0.5 µg/min infusion is used when the serum Cr is > 4 mg/dl. Patients remain on aspirin and heparin.

   Tirofiban (Aggrastat) is given as a 0.4 µg/kg/min infusion for 30 minutes, followed by an infusion of 0.1 µg/kg/min for 48 hours. Like eptifibatide, tirofiban is given with heparin and aspirin.

9. Statin therapy should be started. There are numerous statins to choose from, including atorvastatin (Lipitor) 10 to 20 mg per day, simvastatin (Zocor) 10 to 20 mg per day, and pravastatin (Pravachol) 20 to 40 mg per day.

BIBLIOGRAPHY

Cohn, M., Demers, C., Gurfinkel, E.P., et al. A comparison of low-molecular-weight heparin with unfractioned heparin for unstable coronary artery disease. *N. Engl. J. Med.* 336: 447–452, 1997.

Gurfinkel, E.P., Manos, E.J., Mejaíl, R.I., et al. Low molecular weight heparin versus regular heparin or aspirin in the treatment of unstable angina and silent ischemia. *J. Am. Coll. Cardiol.* 26:313–318, 1995.

Klein, W., Buchwald, A., Hillis, S.E., et al. Comparison of low-molecular-weight heparin with unfractionated heparin acutely and with placebo for 6 weeks in the management of unstable coronary artery disease. *Circulation* 96: 61–68, 1997.

Kontny, F., Dale, J., Abildgaard, U., and Pedersen, T.R. Randomized trial of low molecular weight heparin (Dalteparin) in prevention of left ventricular thrombus formation and arterial embolism after acute anterior myocardial infarction: The Fragmin in Acute Myocardial Infarction (FRAMI) Study. *J. Am. Coll. Cardiol.* 30:962–969, 1997.

Narins, C.R., and Topol, E.J. Attention shifts to the white clot. *Lancet* 2 (suppl III):350, 1997.

PARAGON Investigators. International, randomized, controlled trial of lamifiban (a platelet glycoprotein IIb/IIIa inhibitor), heparin, or both in unstable angina. *Circulation* 97:2386–2395, 1998.

PRISM Study Investigators. A comparison of aspirin plus tirofiban with aspirin plus heparin for unstable angina. *N. Engl. J. Med.* 338:1498–1505, 1998.

PRISM-PLUS Study Investigators. Inhibition of the platelet glycoprotein IIb/IIIa receptor with tirofiban in unstable angina and non-Q-wave myocardial infarction. *N. Engl. J. Med.* 338:1488–1497, 1998.

PURSUIT Trial Investigators. Inhibition of platelet glycoprotein IIb/IIIa with eptifibatide in patients with acute coronary syndromes. *N. Engl. J. Med.* 339:436–443, 1998.

Théroux, P., and Fuster, V. Acute coronary syndromes: Unstable angina and non-Q-wave myocardial infarction. *Circulation* 97:1195–1206, 1998.

Yun, D.D., and Alpert, J.S. Acute coronary syndromes. *Cardiology* 88:223–237, 1997.

24

Treatment of Angina in the Immediate Postinfarction Period

Patients with angina in the immediate (first 3 weeks) postinfarction period should be treated in a manner similar to that employed for patients with unstable angina (see Chapter 23). It is not unusual for patients with acute myocardial infarction (AMI) to have some residual chest discomfort for 2 to 3 days after the acute event. Moreover, a modest number of patients with MI develop early (first 72 hours) or late (7 days to several months) pericarditis (see Chapter 25). Pain from the latter condition can easily be confused with angina pectoris unless the characteristic positional (pain worse on recumbency and improved on sitting) and pleuritic (pain worse on inspiration) qualities of pericarditic discomfort are elicited. Pericardial rubs are usually evanescent, hence the absence of a rub does not rule out the diagnosis of pericarditis. Unstable angina following AMI can develop despite thrombolytic therapy.

PROTOCOL

1. If a patient develops chest discomfort suggestive of myocardial ischemia (at rest or associated with exertion, such as at the morning toilet), if such pain occurs between 2 and 21 days after infarction, and if pericarditis seems unlikely, then it should be assumed that the patient is suffering from angina pectoris immediately after infarction.

2. Signs and symptoms of left ventricular failure should be sought, since a dilated left ventricle with a high filling pressure has a higher myocardial oxygen consumption than the same ventricle at a smaller volume and with a lower filling pressure.

    a. Patients who are felt to have significant left ventricular failure (e.g., rales, S_3; cardiomegaly or pulmonary vascular redistribution by radiograph, elevated filling pressures) should be treated with diuretics, vasodilators, and digitalis, as described in Chapter 19.

    b. If angina still occurs in the absence of adequate treatment for left ventricular failure or following it, then metoprolol or another beta blocker, nitrate, and/or calcium channel blocker should be initiated as described in Chapter 23. All anginal episodes should be promptly treated with sublingual nitroglycerin (with two to three repeated doses if necessary and if the blood pressure is adequate) or even intravenous nitroglycerin, depending on the perceived instability of the patient. Activity should be moderately reduced until adequate beta-blocker and nitrate dosage has been achieved (for example, metoprolol 50 to 100 mg q12h; isosorbide dinitrate 5 to 20 mg chewed or sublingually q2 to 3h; diltiazem 60 mg q8h). Thereafter, activity may be increased again to see if the episodes of angina pectoris recur. Concomitant triple therapy (i.e., beta blockers, nitrates, and calcium channel blockers), intravenous nitroglycerin therapy, or both may be required in recalcitrant cases of postinfarction angina. Aspirin (325 mg PO daily) and intravenous unfractionated or subcutaneous low-molecular-weight heparin should be administered. A modified exercise test is performed on all patients prior to discharge once stability is achieved. Cardiac catheterization should be strongly considered (see paragraph c, below).

c. If angina pectoris recurs with minimal or very modest activity or if the patient has a clearly positive modified exercise test, it is probable that anginal attacks will occur even more frequently at home following discharge from the hospital. Such patients are at high risk for infarct extension. Therefore, cardiac catheterization and coronary artery bypass surgery or coronary angioplasty should be strongly considered (see Chapter 30).

d. Coronary artery surgery is best performed at least 3 to 4 weeks following an acute transmural MI. If angina pectoris can be controlled medically, then surgery can safely be delayed until 4 weeks after infarction. Clearly, many patients will have angina of such a refractory nature that surgery cannot be delayed. The timing of catheterization and surgery in such patients must be individualized.

BIBLIOGRAPHY

Benhorin, J., Andrews, M.L., Carleen, E.D., et al. Occurrence, characteristics, and prognostic significance of early postacute myocardial infarction angina pectoris. *Am. J. Cardiol.* 62:679–685, 1988.

Crea, F., et al. Effects of verapamil in preventing early postinfarction angina and reinfarction. *Am. J. Cardiol.* 55: 900–904, 1985.

Marmor, A., Sobel, B.E., and Roberts, R. Factors presaging early recurrent myocardial infarction ("extension"). *Am. J. Cardiol.* 48:603–610, 1981.

Also see references for Chapter 22.

25

Treatment of Miscellaneous Complications of Acute Myocardial Infarction: Pericarditis, Pulmonary Embolism, Left Ventricular Thrombus, Arterial Embolism, and Myocardial Rupture

PERICARDITIS

Peri-infarction pericarditis is diagnosed by an accurate history. In the past it has probably occurred in about 25% of patients with acute ST-T-wave elevation myocardial infarction (MI) when diagnosed by a careful history and physical exam. The average incidence has been only 14% if one requires the presence of a friction rub. The incidence of peri-infarction pericarditis has been reduced by 50% with thrombolytic therapy, so that only about 15% of patients with acute ST-T-wave elevation MI have a typical history, and only 5% to 7% of patients with MI have an audible pericardial friction rub. Although the frequency of a pericardial function rub is low in the thrombolytic era, its occurrence denotes extensive myocardial damage with a worse outcome. The electrocardiogram (ECG) may show P-R segment depression, persistently elevated T waves for 48 hours or longer after the onset of acute MI (AMI), or initially inverted T waves that become positive. Chest discomfort is pleuritic, usually comes on 2 to 4 days following infarction, and can be accompanied by low-grade fever. The chest discomfort is persistent though sometimes improved by sitting up and leaning forward. It is important to differentiate it from ischemic pain, which is usually an indication for early coronary angiography.

PROTOCOL

1. Ibuprofen 300 to 800 mg every 6 to 8 hours
2. Aspirin 324 to 650 mg every 4 to 6 hours
3. Avoid the use of corticosteroids
4. Avoid anti-coagulation with warfarin

PULMONARY EMBOLISM

It is not clear how often acute pulmonary embolism (PE) occurs in patients with AMI, but it is seemingly not common.

It is the great masquerader and should always be considered in a patient who becomes tachypneic, tachycardic, and hypoxemic. Unexplained weakness, sweating, fever, and dyspnea can also be presenting features. Stasis obesity and immobilization may predispose the patient toward acute PE.

When the diagnosis of PE is clinically suspected, a plasma D-dimer determined by enzyme-linked immunosorbent assay (ELISA) should be ordered. The test is sensitive (90%) but not specific for PE. Arterial blood gases are not always helpful. Echocardiography is a rapid, practical, and sensitive technique. Detection of right ventricular dilation and dysfunction is consistent with acute PE, particularly if the RV hypokinesis spares the apex. A chest x-ray, ECG, and leg ultrasonagraphy should also be considered. A lung scan or spiral computed tomography should be considered in cases of intermediate probability. A normal lung scan essentially excludes PE. If these tests are unrevealing, pulmonary angiography should be considered. The standard treatment for pulmonary embolus is heparin, though treatment with thrombolysis or mechanical intervention is used if the patient is hemodynamocally unstable. Temporary mechanical ventilation for hypoxemia and dobutamine for hypotension are useful adjunctive measures.

PROTOCOL

1. Heparin in a bolus of 80 U/kg followed by 18 U/kg/h to keep a PTT at 46 to 70 seconds. Heparin infusion rates as high as 1500 to 2000 U/h are quite commonly required to achieve adequate anti-coagulation during the first few days of heparin administration. Heparin is continued for 5 to 7 days. Low-molecular-weight heparin may be just as effective. Warfarin is usually given for at least 3 months.

2. When warfarin is initiated (5 mg/day), it should overlap with heparin for 5 days. Target INR = 2.0 to 3.0.

3. When there is hemodynamic compromise, tissue plasminogen activator (t-PA) should be considered. Give 100 mg as a continuous peripheral intravenous infusion administered over 2 hours, followed by intravenous heparin.

4. If there is failed thrombolysis, a contraindication for thrombolysis, or hemodynamic compromise, pulmonary embolectomy in the cath lab or operating room should be considered.

LEFT VENTRICULAR THROMBUS
AND ARTERIAL EMBOLISM

The current prevalence of LV thrombus in anterior wall AMI by echocardiography is lower than previously reported, perhaps owing to thrombolytic therapy. The prevalence is 0.6% at day 1, 3.7% at day 14, and 2.5% at day 90 post-MI. Resolution documented by echocardiography is frequent. A decreased ejection fraction and older age predispose to stroke. Acute and chronic anticoagulation with warfarin is given to prevent further thrombus formation and reduce the incidence of systemic embolization. Peripheral arterial emboli to an extremity represent an emergency, and such patients should be examined as soon as possible by a vascular surgeon. Embolectomy is usually indicated.

PROTOCOL

1. For LV thrombus noted after AMI, start full-dose heparin and continue for 5 to 7 days to keep aPTT 46 to 70 seconds.
    Start warfarin 5 mg/day PO to overlap with heparin for 3 to 5 days. Target INR = 2.0 to 3.0. Continue warfarin for 3 to 6 months. Thrombus may resolve sooner.
2. For arterial embolus to an extremity, start full-dose heparin at once; contact vascular surgeons ASAP for possible embolectomy.

MYOCARDIAL RUPTURE

Myocardial rupture is a catastrophic event that occurs suddenly in 10% to 15% of patients with AMI. It usually occurs in the first week and is more common in elderly hypertensive women. It may occur earlier (<48 hours) in the thrombolytic era. Death usually occurs within minutes and is heralded by cardiovascular collapse and electromechanical dissociation, bradycardia, and asystole. Rarely, patients survive long enough to be brought to the operating room, where the defect can be closed.

BIBLIOGRAPHY

Becker, R.C., Gore, J.M., Lambrew, C.T., et al. A composite view of cardiac rupture in the United States national registry of myocardial infarction. *J. Am. Coll. Cardiol.* 27: 1321–1326, 1996.

Becker, R.C., Hochman, J.S., Cannon, C.P., et al. Fatal cardiac rupture among patients treated with thrombolytic agents and adjunctive thrombin antagonists. *J. Am. Coll. Cardiol.* 33:479–487, 1999.

Daniels, L.B., Parker, A., Patel, S.R., Grodstein, F., and Goldhaber, S.Z. Relation of duration of symptoms with response to thrombolytic therapy in pulmonary embolism. *Am. J. Cardiol.* 80:184–188, 1997.

Goldhaber, S.Z. Pulmonary embolism. *N. Engl. J. Med.* 339: 93–104, 1998.

Greaves, S.C., Zhi, G., Lee, R.T., et al. Incidence and natural history of left ventricular thrombus following anterior wall acute myocardial infarction. *Am. J. Cardiol.* 80: 442–448, 1997.

Kasper, W., Konstantinides, S., Geibel, A., et al. Management strategies and determinants of outcome in acute major pulmonary embolism: Results of a multicenter registry. *J. Am. Coll. Cardiol.* 30:1165–1173, 1997.

Keeley, E.C., and Hillis, L.D. Left ventricular mural thrombus after acute myocardial infarction. *Clin. Cardiol.* 19: 83–86, 1996.

Loh, E., Martin, Sutton, M. St. J., Wun, C.C., et al. Ventricular dysfunction and the risk of stroke after myocardial infarction. *N. Engl. J. Med.* 336:251–257, 1997.

Olivia, P.B., Hammill, C., and Talano, J.V. Effect of definition on incidence of postinfarction pericarditis. Is it time to redefine postinfarction pericarditis? *Circulation.* 90: 1537–1541, 1994.

Sajadieh, A., Wendelboe, O., Fischer Hansen, J., and Spang Mortensen, L. Nonsteroidal anti-inflammatory drugs after acute myocardial infarction. *Am. J. Cardiol.* 83:1263–1264, 1999.

Simonneau, G., Sors, H., and Charbonnier, B. A comparison of low-molecular weight heparin for acute pulmonary embolism. *N. Engl. J. Med.* 337:663–669, 1997.

Tofler, G.H., Muller, J.E., and Stone, P.H. Pericarditis in acute myocardial infarction: Characterization and clinical significance. Am. Heart J. 117:86–90, 1989.

Wall, T.C., Califf, R.M., and Harrelson-Woodlief, L. Usefulness of a pericardial friction rub after thrombolytic therapy during acute myocardial infarction in predicting amount of myocardial damage. *Am. J. Cardiol.* 66:1418–1421, 1990.

Wells, P.S., Ginsberg, J.S., and Anderson, D.R. Use of a clinical model for safe management of patients with suspected pulmonary embolism. *Ann. Intern. Med.* 129:997–1011, 1998.

26

Diagnosis and Treatment of Right Ventricular Infarction

Once thought to be rare, infarction of the right ventricular myocardium is now known to occur in approximately 30% of patients with Q-wave inferior infarction. In most patients, the volume of right ventricular myocardium that is infarcted is small, and thus these patients rarely develop signs or symptoms of right ventricular failure. However, modest right ventricular dysfunction can be demonstrated in many patients with transmural inferior infarction by means of noninvasive cardiac diagnostic techniques (echocardiography, radionuclide angiocardiography). The diagnosis is suggested if ST-segment elevation is present in the right precordial leads (Tables 26-1 and 26-2). Right ventricular infarction is associated with a significant (25% to 30%) increase in hospital mortality.

Occasional patients with acute inferior wall myocardial infarction (MI) present with severe right ventricular failure and hypotension, which suggests that extensive right ventricular infarction has occurred. Noninvasive cardiac evaluation often demonstrates near-normal left ventricular function and marked right ventricular dysfunction in such patients.

A distinct hemodynamic pattern that can mimic cardiac tamponade or constrictive pericarditis is seen in patients with predominant right ventricular infarction. Volume expansion therapy alone may be successful in the treatment of low cardiac output and hypotension resulting from predominant right ventricular infarction. Other patients with right ventricular infarction develop refractory hypotension and for them more aggressive management is indicated. Successful thrombolytic therapy can rapidly reverse the clinical syndrome of right ventricular infarction.

PROTOCOL
1. The diagnosis of predominant right ventricular infarction is entertained in patients with Q-wave inferior MI who develop hypotension and jugular venous distention, usually in the absence of pulmonary congestion. Right precordial lead electrocardiographic tracings frequently demonstrate ST-segment elevation in patients with right ventricular infarction.

**Table 26-1. Diagnostic features
of right ventricular infarction**

Procedure	Findings
History	Symptoms of acute MI
Physical examination	Hypotension
	Pulsus paradoxus (±)
	Distended neck veins
	Kussmaul's sign
	Clear lungs
	RV S_3 and S_4
	Tricuspid insufficiency murmur (±)
	Hepatic tenderness (±)
Laboratory studies	Electrocardiogram
	Acute inferior or posterior MI
	ST-segment elevation (occasionally depression) in right-sided precordial leads
	Bradycardia, A-V block, ventricular arrhythmias
	Chest roentgenogram
	Clear lung fields
	Echocardiogram
	Dilated hypokinetic RV
	Segmental RV wall motion abnormalities
	Absence of large pericardial effusion
	Paradoxical ventricular septal motion
	Tricuspid insufficiency
	RVG
	Dilated RV
	Depressed RV systolic function
	Regional RV wall motion abnormalities
	Decreased LV/RV stroke volume ratio
	Increased RV/LV area ratio
	Technetium pyrophosphate scan
	Isotope uptake in the RV free wall, septum, and posterior LV
	Thallium-201 scintigraphy
	Decreased uptake in the RV septum, and posterior LV
	Cardiac catheterization and bedside hemodynamic monitoring
	Occluded RCA (occasionally left circumflex in left dominant system)
	Equalization of diastolic pressures during right heart catheterization
	Low PA systolic pressure
	Diastolic dip-and-plateau in RV
	V wave in RA if tricuspid insufficiency present
	In RA $y > x$

A-V, atrioventricular; LV, left ventricle; MI, myocardial infarction; PA, pulmonary artery; RCA, right coronary artery; RV, right ventricle; RVG, radionuclide ventriculogram; RA, right atrial pressure curve.
(From Barnard D, Alpert JS. Right ventricular infarction. In: Rippe JM, Irwin RS, Alpert JS, Dalen JE, eds. *Intensive Care Medicine,* 2nd ed. Boston: Little, Brown, 1991. With permission.)

a.   Confirmation of the diagnosis is obtained by means of echocardiography (increased right ventricular end-diastolic dimension and decreased right ventricular systolic function), radionuclide angiocardiography (decreased ejection fraction and increased volume of the right ventricle), or right heart catheterization (see paragraph b, below).

b.   Further confirmation of the diagnosis and a guide to therapy can be obtained, if clinically indicated by patient instability, by means of a right heart catheterization with a flow-directed balloon-tipped catheter. Hemodynamic findings in predominant right ventricular infarction can include the following: elevated right atrial and right ventricular end-diastolic pressure that is equal to or greater than pulmonary arterial or pulmonary capillary wedge pressure; normal pulmonary arterial systolic pressure; normal pulmonary vascular resistance; pulsus paradoxus greater than 10 mm Hg in the arterial pressure; and occasionally an inspiratory increase in right atrial pressure (Kussmaul's sign). The latter two findings, together with equalization of end-diastolic right heart pressures (right atrial, right ventricular, pulmonary arterial, and pulmonary capillary wedge) may suggest the erroneous diagnosis of cardiac constriction or compression. Echocardiographic and radionuclide angiocardiographic examination of right ventricular function can usually distinguish right ventricular infarction from cardiac tamponade or constrictive pericarditis (see Table 26-1). Elevated right atrial pressure may suggest acute pulmonary embolism (see chapter 25). Normal pulmonary arterial pressure and, if necessary, normal perfusion on a pulmonary scintigram rule out pulmonary embolism (see Table 26-2).

2.   Patients who meet the criteria that have been outlined for predominant right ventricular infarction are managed as follows:

a.   In the absence of hypotension and severe bradyarrhythmias, patients are managed expectantly.

b.   If hypotension is present, bradyarrhythmias or atrial fibrillation should be corrected as outlined in Chapter 17. An occasional patient with right ventricular infarction and bradyarrhythmias refractory to atropine administration, as well as hypotension

Table 26-2. Differential diagnosis of right ventricular infarction

Procedure	RVI	Cardiac Tamponade	Pulmonary Embolism	Constrictive Pericardial Disease	Restrictive Cardiomyopathy
History	Symptoms of acute MI	Symptoms of underlying diseases	Pleuritic chest pain, dyspnea, predisposing factors	Symptoms of underlying diseases	Symptoms of underlying diseases
Physical examination	Hypotension Pulsus paradoxus Jugular venous distention Kussmaul's sign Clear lungs RV S_3 and S_4 Tricuspid insufficiency murmur Hepatic tenderness	Hypotension Pulsus paradoxus Jugular venous distention Muffled heart sounds	Hypotension Pulsus paradoxus Jugular venous distention Kussmaul's sign Tachypnea Loud P_2 Widely split second heart sound	Friedreich's sign Jugular venous distention Pericardial knock Ascites with lower extremity edema	Kussmaul's sign Friedreich's sign ± Pulsus paradoxus Biventricular S_3 and S_4 Rales
Laboratory findings	MI enzyme pattern S-T elevation right precordial leads		Room-air blood gases: hypoxemia and acute respiratory alkalosis		

Chest roentgenogram	Clear lung fields Late right pleural effusion	Large bottle-shaped heart	Pleural effusion Infiltrate	Pericardial calcification Pleural thickening or effusion Signs of TB	Cardiomegaly Pulmonary venous congestion
Electrocardiogram	Inferior, posterior MI S-T elevation right precordial leads	Low voltage	p-Pulmonale Right axis deviation S_1, Q_3, T_3	Nonspecific S-T and T wave changes Increased incidence of atrial fibrillation	Low voltage conduction defects
Echocardiogram	Dilated, hypokinetic RV Segmental wall motion abnormalities in RV	Pericardial effusion Small, hyperdynamic ventricle (LV, RV)	Dilated RV Global RV dysfunction	Pericardial effusion Small, vigorously contracting ventricle (LV, RV)	Diastolic dysfunction Ventricular contraction may be normal With amyloid, myocardial speckling and increased mass

continued

Table 26-2. *Continued*

Procedure	RVI	Cardiac Tamponade	Pulmonary Embolism	Constrictive Pericardial Disease	Restrictive Cardiomyopathy
Radionuclide ventriculogram	Dilated, hypokinetic RV; segmental wall motion abnormalities				
Pyrophosphate scintigram	Uptake RV, septum, LV inferior wall				With amyloid, diffuse uptake
Cardiac catheterization and bedside hemodynamic monitoring	Equalization of diastolic pressures Diastolic dip-and-plateau in RV tracing $y = x$ or $y > x$ in RA tracing V waves in RA if tricuspid insufficiency murmur present	Equalization of diastolic pressures Increased RA pressure Decreased y descent	Elevated RA pressure with normal waves Elevated PA systolic pressure Gradient from PA diastolic to PCW pressure	Equalization of diastolic pressures RA tracing flat RV dip-and-plateau	Equalization of diastolic pressures RA with prominent x and y RV dip-and-plateau

| Other diagnostic modalities | Elevated RA relative to PCW pressure | Ventilation-perfusion scan Pulmonary arteriogram abnormal Impedance plethysmography abnormal | Computed tomography abnormal |

RV, right ventricle; LV, left ventricle; RA, right atrium; PCW, pulmonary capillary wedge; PA, pulmonary artery. (From Barnard, D, Alpert, JS. Right ventricular infarction. In Rippe JM, Irwin RS, Alpert JS, and Dalen JE, eds. *Intensive Care Medicine*, 2nd ed. Boston: Little, Brown, 1991. With permission.)

may respond rapidly to atrioventricular (A-V) sequential pacing. Ventricular pacing alone is usually unsuccessful in reversing hypotension in these individuals if A-V block is present. Intravascular volume expansion with dextran or colloid solutions should be undertaken. Volume expansion should be continued until right atrial pressure reaches a level of at least 14 to 15 mm Hg (often, higher pressures are required to reverse systemic hypotension).

c. If hypotension persists after correction of bradyarrhythmias and plasma volume expansion, dopamine or dobutamine infusion is indicated (Chapter 19). Intra-aortic balloon counterpulsation has also been employed on occasion in these patients, but it is unclear whether this intervention is beneficial in those with predominant right ventricular infarction.

d. Successful pharmacologic or mechanical thrombolytic therapy can reverse the signs of right ventricular infarction. Such therapy must be initiated as soon as possible after the onset of infarction (see Chapter 13).

e. If systemic arterial pressure is adequate but signs and symptoms of marked right ventricular failure develop (hepatic congestion with rising serum enzymes and bilirubin, low cardiac output with rising blood urea nitrogen), patients may be treated with simultaneous infusions of nitroprusside (see Chapter 19) and plasma volume expanders. Angiotensin-converting enzyme (ACE) inhibition may be employed with careful attention paid to renal function.

BIBLIOGRAPHY

Andersen, H.R., Falk, E., and Nielsen, D. Right ventricular infarction: Frequency, size and topography in coronary heart disease: A prospective study comprising 107 consecutive autopsies from a coronary care unit. *J. Am. Coll. Cardiol.* 10:1223–1232, 1987.

Baigrie, R.S., et al. The spectrum of right ventricular involvement in inferior wall myocardial infarction: A clinical, hemodynamic, and noninvasive study. *J. Am. Coll. Cardiol.* 6:1396–1404, 1983.

Bellamy, G.R., Rasmussen, H.H., Nasser, F.N., Wiseman, J.C., and Cooper, R.A. Value of two-dimensional echocardiography, electrocardiography, and clinical signs in detecting right ventricular infarction. *Am. Heart J.* 112: 304–309, 1986.

Berger, P.B., Ruocco, N.A. Jr., Ryan, T.J., et al. Frequency and significance of right ventricular dysfunction during inferior wall left ventricular myocardial infarction treated with thrombolytic therapy [results from the thrombolysis in myocardial infarction (TIMI) II trial]: The TIMI Research Group. *Am. J. Cardiol.* 71:1148–1152, 1993.

Bowers, T.R., O'Neill, W.W., Grines, C., Pica, M.C., Safian, R.D., and Goldstein, J.A. Effect of reperfusion on biventricular function and survival after right ventricular infarction. *N. Engl. J. Med.* 338:933–940, 1998.

Chou, T.C., Van der Bel-Kahn, J., Allen, J., Brockmeier, L., and Fowler, N.O. Electrocardiographic diagnosis of right ventricular infarction. *Am. J. Med.* 70:1175–1180, 1981.

Cintron, G.B., Hernandez, E., Linares, E., and Aranda, J.M. Bedside recognition, incidence and clinical course of right ventricular infarction. *Am. J. Cardiol.* 47:224–227, 1981.

Cohn, J.N., Guiha, N.H., Broder, M.I., and Limas, C.J. Right ventricular infarction. *Am. J. Cardiol.* 33:209–214, 1974.

Croft, C.H., Nicod, P., Corbett, J.R., et al. Detection of acute right ventricular infarction by right precordial electrocardiography. *Am. J. Cardiol.* 50:421–427, 1982.

Dell'Italia, L.J., et al. Comparative effects of volume loading, dobutamine, and nitroprusside in patients with predominant right ventricular infarction. *Circulation* 72:1327–1335, 1985.

Goldstein, J.A., Barzilai, B., Rosmond, T.L., Eisenberg, P.R., and Jaffe, A.S. Determinants of hemodynamic compromise with severe right ventricular infarction. *Circulation* 82:359–368, 1990.

Jensen, D.P., Goolsby, J.P., Jr., and Oliva, P.B. Hemodynamic pattern resembling pericardial constriction after acute inferior myocardial infarction with right ventricular infarction. *Am. J. Cardiol.* 42:858–861, 1978.

Kinch, J.W., and Ryan, T.J. Right ventricular infarction. *N. Engl. J. Med.* 330:1211–1217, 1994.

Klein, H.O., Tordjman, T., Ninio, R., et al. The early recognition of right ventricular infarction: Diagnostic accuracy of the electrocardiographic V_4R lead. *Circulation* 67: 558–565, 1983.

Love, J.C., Haffajee, C.I., Gore, J.M., and Alpert, J.S. Reversibility of hypotension and shock by atrial or atrioventricular sequential pacing in patients with right ventricular infarction. *Am. Heart J.* 108:5–13, 1984.

Rackley, C.E., Russell, R.O., Jr., Mantle, J.A., Rogers, W.J., Papapietro, S.E., and Schwartz, K.M. Right ventricular infarction and function. *Am. Heart J.* 101:215–218, 1981.

Robalino, B.D., Whitlow, P.L., Underwood, D.A., and Salcedo, E.E. Electrocardiographic manifestations of right ventricular infarction. *Am. Heart J.* 118:138–144, 1989.

Sugiura, T., Iwasaka, T., Takahashi, N., et al. Atrial fibrillation in inferior wall Q-wave acute myocardial infarction. *Am. J. Cardiol.* 67:1135–1136, 1991.

Williams, J.F. Right ventricular infarction. *Clin. Cardiol.* 13:309–315, 1990.

Yasuda, T., Okada, R.D., Leinbach, R.C., et al. Serial evaluation of right ventricular dysfunction associated with acute inferior myocardial infarction. *Am. Heart J.* 119:816–822, 1990.

Zehender, M., Kasper, W., Kauder, E., et al. Right ventricular infarction as an independent predictor of prognosis after acute inferior myocardial infarction. *N. Engl. J. Med.* 328:981–988, 1993.

27

Electrical Cardioversion: Indications and Procedure

Cardioversion is a dramatic form of therapy that can quickly restore circulatory integrity and is often lifesaving. The sooner electrical defibrillation is initiated, the greater the success rate. The technical aspects of cardioversion are quite important. The electrodes are placed anteriorly over the sternum or just next to the sternum at the third intercoastal space. Firm pressure is applied. The second electrode is placed posteriorly just below the left scapula, with generous amounts of gel. The second paddle is usually placed to the left of the nipple in the mid-axillary line. Once the desired energy level is selected, a second switch is used to charge the capacitor. For atrial fibrillation, 200 J is given, while 50 J is used initially for supraventriclar tachycardia (SVT) or atrial flutter. The patient should be sedated and the shock synchronized with the electrocardiographic QRS complex.

For ventricular fibrillation, the initial shock should be 200 J. The strength of the second shock should be 300 J. Cardiac arrest victims in ventricular fibrillation should undergo at least three attempts at external defibrillation as the initial step to resuscitation. Hemodynamically stable ventricular tachycardia can frequently be cardioverted with 30 to 50 J. Hemodynamically unstable patients or patients with myocardial ischemia require urgent cardioversion, and there is no time to ensure adequate anticoagulation.

Elective cardioversion for atrial fibrillation or atrial flutter of recent onset (48 hours or less) should be performed with full-dose heparin on board. If heparin is contraindicated, a transesophageal echocardiogram (TEE) should be done looking for intra-cardiac clot. If the TEE is negative, cardioversion can be attempted, but even a negative TEE does not preclude the occurrence of a cerebral embolus. Even patients undergoing chemical cardioversion should be anticoagulated. If a clot is identified by TEE, anticoagulation for at least 6 weeks prior to repeat TEE and cardioversion, and for 3 to 6 months after cardioversion is recommended. Cardioversion is considered only if the TEE is negative for clots.

PROTOCOL
1. For emergencies (e.g., ventricular fibrillation or hemodynamically unstable ventricular tachycardia), immedi-

ate cardioversion is indicated. Cardiovert with 200 J, followed by 300 and 360 J if necessary.

2. For atrial fibrillation of less than 48 hours duration, give full-dose heparin; sedate patient with short-acting barbituate (e.g., methohexital or Brevital) or etomidate with anesthesiology standby. Cardiovert with 200 J after synchronizing to electrocardiographic (ECG) QRS.

3. For atrial flutter persisting for less than 48 hours, give full-dose heparin; sedate patient; synchronize to ECG; and cardiovert with 50 J.

4. For elective cardioversion when duration of rhythm is uncertain, anticoagulate with heparin and warfarin. Continue warfarin for 3 to 6 weeks prior to cardioversion, and for 1 to 3 months after cardioversion. If the duration of the rhythm is less than 6 weeks but greater than 48 hours, consider TEE; if TEE is negative, proceed with cardioversion after 2 days of heparin.

5. There is always a chance that systemic embolism and stroke may occur after cardioversion, electrical or chemical. A negative TEE does not predict complete absence of post-cardioversion embolus. In general, anticoagulation prior to and after cardioversion is indicated for most patients. If anticoagulation is contraindicated (e.g., active bleeding), consider TEE. If the TEE is negative, proceed with cardioversion.

BIBLIOGRAPHY

Ewy, G.A. Optimal technique for electrical cardioversion of atrial fibrillation. *Circulation* 86: 1645–1647, 1992.

Kowey, P.R. The calamity of cardioversion of conscious patients. *Am. J. Cardiol.* 61: 1106–1107, 1988.

Prystowsky, E.N., Benson, W., Fuster, V., et al. Management of patients with atrial fibrillation. *Circulation* 93: 1262–1277, 1996.

Silverman, D.I., and Manning, W.J. Role of echocardiography in patients undergoing elective cardioversion of atrial fibrillation. *Circulation* 98: 479–486, 1998.

Weigner, M.J., Caulfield, T.A., Danias, P.G., Silverman, D.I., and Manning, W.J. Risk for clinical thromboembolism associated with conversion to sinus rhythm in patients with atrial fibrillation lasting less than 48 hours. *Ann. Intern. Med* 126: 615–620, 1997.

28

Counterpulsation in Patients with Myocardial Infarction or Unstable Angina: Indications and Procedure

Counterpulsation is a technique whereby the volume of blood in the aorta is transiently increased during diastole by means of a mechanical device. This sudden increase in aortic diastolic volume results in an increase in aortic diastolic pressure.

Most of left ventricular myocardial blood flow occurs during diastole. Hence, increased aortic diastolic blood pressure results in a greater perfusion pressure for the coronary bed during diastole. This increased perfusion pressure forces more blood through a stenotic coronary arterial system and thus increases myocardial blood flow in patients with coronary artery disease. It is obvious that increased myocardial blood flow benefits the patient with critical myocardial ischemia.

Moreover, rapid deflation of the intra-aortic balloon (the most common form of counterpulsation is performed with an intra-aortic balloon) at the onset of left ventricular systole leads to a decrease in aortic systolic pressure. This decrease in systemic arterial pressure reduces left ventricular work in a manner comparable to that obtained with arterial vasodilator drugs (i.e., afterload-reducing agents such as nitroprusside). The result of such afterload reduction is an increase in cardiac output. Thus, counterpulsation (particularly intra-aortic balloon counterpulsation) has two beneficial effects on the left ventricle: (a) left ventricular myocardial blood flow is increased and (b) left ventricular work is reduced, leading to an increase in cardiac output.

Two forms of counterpulsation are available. Internal or balloon counterpulsation requires the placement of an elongated, sausage-shaped balloon in the descending aorta. The balloon is inserted percutaneously like a cardiac catheter or through a tubular Dacron graft side arm sewn into the patient's femoral artery. The balloon, triggered by the electrocardiogram (ECG), is rapidly inflated with CO_2 or helium during cardiac diastole, thus transiently increasing aortic volume and pressure. This is the most common form of counterpulsation.

External counterpulsation involves surrounding the patient's lower extremities (from ankle to upper thigh) with plastic leggings. The water or air pressure within these leggings is increased to 150 to 200 mm Hg during cardiac diastole. This external compression of the legs forces arterial blood back into the aorta and venous blood forward into the vena cava. Thus, diastolic aortic and vena caval volume and pressure increase, resulting in simultaneous increases in ventricular filling and myocardial blood flow.

Both forms of counterpulsation are effective in supporting the circulation of animals with experimental cardiogenic shock and of patients with that clinical entity. Moreover, there is evidence that counterpulsation reduces experimental infarct size in animals, and morbidity and mortality in patients with myocardial infarction (MI) and left ventricular failure (see Chapter 12). Internal or balloon counterpulsation affords greater hemodynamic support than does external counterpulsation. Therefore, intra-aortic balloon counterpulsation is the technique employed to support patients with cardiogenic shock.

Current indications for counterpulsation include (a) cardiogenic shock (see Chapter 21) secondary to MI or following cardiac surgery; (b) highly unstable angina pectoris (see Chapter 23); and (c) severe left ventricular failure with or without acute mitral regurgitation or ventricular septal rupture (see Chapter 20). The combination of counterpulsation and afterload reduction with nitroprusside (see Chapter 19) has been shown to be particularly effective in selected patients with severe left ventricular failure. Counterpulsation is contraindicated in patients with aortic dissection, large aortic aneurysms, aortic regurgitation, and severe peripheral vascular disease.

The application and correct use of counterpulsation devices require training. This procedure should be performed by a knowledgeable team that can be rapidly mobilized at any time. The insertion of the aortic balloon is usually performed by a cardiologist or a thoracic or vascular surgeon. In the case of a patient felt to be a candidate for counterpulsation, Cardiac Surgery should be consulted. It is particularly important to consult Cardiac Surgery in such cases, because patients who require counterpulsation rarely survive for more than a few days or weeks without a definitive surgical procedure (i.e., coronary artery bypass, mitral valve replacement, closure of a ventricular septal defect, or aneurysmectomy) (see Chapter 30). Counterpulsation can also be employed to stabilize patients following coronary angioplasty.

PROTOCOL

1. Protocols for patients on intra-aortic balloon counterpulsation vary from hospital to hospital. The following is a typical (but not the only possible) protocol for such patients:

   a. The clinical and hemodynamic signs to be monitored hourly include intra-arterial blood pressure, pulmonary arterial and pulmonary capillary wedge pressure (optional), central venous pressure, respiratory rate, heart rate, urine output (in patients with a Foley catheter in place), and pedal pulses.

   b. Temperature is recorded q4h.

   c. The patient is placed on the balloon with 1:1 counterpulsation setting.

   d. Fluid balance: Daily weights are taken; intake and output are recorded each hour.

   e. The arterial line is flushed continuously or intermittently (see Chapter 29).

   f. When employed, the pulmonary arterial line is flushed continuously or intermittently (see Chapter 29).

   g. For other orders regarding the intravenous line, see Chapter 8.

   h. Medications:

      (1) Cephalothin (or other antistaphylococcal antibiotic) is administered intravenously at a dose of 1 g q6h for 48 hours after the initial dose (a total of eight doses).

      (2) Systemic anticoagulation with continuous or intermittent intravenous unfractionated heparin should be provided (see Chapter 14). Some centers administer low-molecular-weight dextran concomitantly.

   i. Laboratory studies:

      (1) Daily blood studies should include blood urea nitrogen, creatinine, electrolytes (may be determined more frequently), complete blood count with differential, prothrombin time, partial thromboplastin time, and platelet count.

      (2) Daily ECGs should be obtained.

      (3) A chest radiograph should be obtained immediately after insertion of the intra-aortic balloon and daily thereafter.

      (4) Daily cultures of the wound at the balloon insertion site are required.

  j. Blood should be typed and held for possible transfusion.

  k. Arterial blood gases should be determined q12h unless the patient is very stable (more often if deemed necessary).

  l. Supplemental inspiratory oxygen should be provided (see Chapter 10).

  m. Chest physiotherapy should be given at least twice daily.

  n. Diet. The patient is kept NPO for 2 to 4 hours after balloon insertion. This is followed by the diet described in Chapter 6. Fluid restriction depends on intake and output and the patient's clinical status.

  o. Activity. The patient is kept on bed rest with the head of the bed elevated not more than 30°. Marked hip flexion should be prevented.

  p. The dressing over the insertion site should be changed daily, with daily application of bactericidal ointment (e.g., povidone-iodine ointment) to the balloon insertion site.

2. A typical protocol for weaning the patient from intra-aortic balloon counterpulsation is as follows:

  a. Intra-aortic balloon weaning settings if tolerated:

      (1) 1:2 for the first 8 hours

      (2) 1:4 for the next 8 hours

      (3) 1:8 for the next 8 hours

Some centers wean patients by gradually decreasing balloon volume but continuing 1:1 counterpulsation.

  b. The following measurements should be recorded after each change in the balloon timing q5min for a total of 15 minutes (three times): blood pressure, heart and respiratory rate, central venous pressure, pulmonary arterial pressure (optional), pulmonary capillary wedge pressure (optional), and urine output. Then they should be recorded q15min for a total of 45 minutes (three times). Then hourly determinations should be resumed after each change in balloon timing (see paragraph a, above).

  c. Arterial blood gases should be determined before weaning begins and after each change in balloon timing (see paragraph a).

  d. The availability of the patient's cross match in the blood bank is checked before removal of the balloon.

e. Intravenous cephalothin (or other antistaphylo-coccal antibiotic), 1 g, is administered 30 minutes before balloon removal and then q6h for a total of eight doses (48 hours).

f. The physician should be notified if any of the following occurs (grounds for discontinuing weaning):
   (1) Hypertension or hypotension
   (2) Rising pulmonary arterial, pulmonary capillary wedge, or central venous pressure
   (3) Diminished urine output
   (4) Change in mental status
   (5) ST-T changes in the 12-lead or monitor-lead ECG
   (6) Chest discomfort
   (7) Change in heart rate, or rhythm, or both, especially if the number of ectopic beats is increased

g. The peripheral pulses should be checked immediately before and after removal of the balloon: q15min for 1 hour (four times) and then qh for 3 hours (three times).

BIBLIOGRAPHY

Amsterdam, E.A., Banas, J., Criley, J.M., et al. Clinical assessment of external pressure circulatory assistance in acute myocardial infarction—Report of a cooperative clinical trial. *Am. J. Cardiol.* 45:349–356, 1980.

Ehrich, D.A., Biddle, T.L., Kronenberg, M.W., and Yu, P.N. The hemodynamic response to intra-aortic balloon counterpulsation in patients with cardiogenic shock complicating acute myocardial infarction. *Am. Heart J.* 93:274–279, 1977.

Flaherty, J.T., Becker, L.C., Weiss, J.L., et al. Results of a randomized prospective trial of intraaortic balloon counterpulsation and intravenous nitroglycerin in patients with acute myocardial infarction. *J. Am. Coll. Cardiol.* 6:434–446, 1985.

Fuchs, R.M., et al. Augmentation of regional coronary blood flow by intra-aortic balloon counterpulsation in patients with unstable angina. *Circulation* 68:117–123, 1983.

Goldberg, M.J., Rubenfire, M., Kantrowitz, A., et al. Intra-aortic balloon pump insertion: A randomized study comparing percutaneous and surgical techniques. *J. Am. Coll. Cardiol.* 9:515–523, 1987.

Gottlieb, S.O., et al. Identification of patients at high-risk for complications of intra-aortic balloon counterpulsation: A multivariate risk factor analysis. *Am. J. Cardiol.* 53: 1135–1139, 1984.

Isner, I.M., Cohen, S.R., Viramani, R., Lawrinson, W., and Roberts, W.C. Complications of the intra-aortic balloon counterpulsation device: Clinical and morphologic observations in 45 necropsy patients. *Am. J. Cardiol.* 45: 260–268, 1980.

Ohman, E.M., Califf, R.M., George, B.S., et al. The use of intraaortic balloon pumping as an adjunct to reperfusion therapy in acute myocardial infarction: The Thrombolysis and Angioplasty in Myocardial Infarction (TAMI) Study Group. *Am. Heart J.* 121:895–901, 1991.

Ohman, E.M., George, B.S., White, C.J., et al. and the Randomized IABP Study Group. Use of aortic counterpulsation to improve sustained coronary artery patency during acute myocardial infarction: Results of a randomized trial. *Circulation* 90:792–799, 1994.

O'Rourke, M.F., Norris, R.M., Campbell, R.J., Chang, V.P., and Sammel, N.L. Randomized controlled trial of intra-aortic balloon counterpulsation in early myocardial infarction with acute heart failure. *Am. J. Cardiol.* 47:815–820, 1981.

Port, S.C., Patel, S., and Schmidt, D.H. Effects of intra-aortic balloon counterpulsation on myocardial blood flow in patients with severe coronary artery disease. *J. Am. Coll. Cardiol.* 3:1367–1374, 1984.

Scheidt, S., Wilner, G., Mueller, H., et al. Intra-aortic balloon counterpulsation in cardiogenic shock: Report of cooperative clinical trial. *N. Engl. J. Med.* 288:979–984, 1973.

Wasfie, T., Freed, P.S., Rubenfire, M, et al. Risks associated with intra-aortic balloon pumping in patients with and without diabetes mellitus. *Am. J. Cardiol.* 61:558–562, 1988.

Weber, K.T., and Janicki, J.S. Intraaortic balloon counterpulsation: A review of physiologic principles, clinical results and device safety. *Ann. Thorac. Surg.* 17:602–636, 1994.

Weiss, A.T., et al. Regional and global left ventricular function during intra-aortic balloon counterpulsation in patients with acute myocardial shock. *Am. Heart J.* 108:249–254, 1984.

Willerson, J.T., Curry, G.C., Watson, J.T., et al. Intra-aortic balloon counterpulsation in patients in cardiogenic shock, medically refractory left ventricular failure and/or recurrent ventricular tachycardia. *Am. J. Med.* 58:183–191, 1975.

Williams, D.O., Korr, K.S., Gewirtz, H., and Most, A.S. The effect of intra-aortic balloon counterpulsation on regional myocardial blood flow and oxygen consumption in the presence of coronary artery stenosis in patients with unstable angina. *Circulation* 66:593–597, 1982.

29

Flow-Directed Catheter Insertion, Arterial Line Insertion, and Interpretation of Data

Hemodynamic measurements made in patients soon after hospitalization for acute myocardial infarction (AMI) usually demonstrate elevated left ventricular end-diastolic pressures (LVEDP). It has generally been accepted that this increase in LVEDP shortly after AMI is due to an increase in stiffness (decreased compliance) of the left ventricle but may also result from an increase in left ventricular end-diastolic volume (Starling mechanism).

Elevations of LVEDP are transmitted to the left atrium and thence to the pulmonary capillaries (normal LVEDP = 3 to 12 mm Hg; normal pulmonary capillary wedge pressure = 1 to 10 mm Hg). Marked elevation of LVEDP, and hence of pulmonary capillary wedge pressure (PCWP), can result in interstitial and eventually alveolar pulmonary edema (at wedge pressures >25 mm Hg). Clinical observations have documented that Starling's law operates in patients with AMI: increases in LVEDP result in increases in cardiac output until a plateau is reached. Pulmonary artery (PA) catheterization with a flow-directed balloon catheter in patients with AMI allows one to estimate a Starling curve for each patient catheterized. Cardiac output is determined by the Fick principle, by dye, or by thermal indicator dilution curves, while LVEDP is gauged from the PCWP. A PCWP of 15 to 18 mm Hg results in optimal cardiac output in most patients with AMI.

Although an attempt should be made to identify A, C, and V waves in the PCWP tracing, this is not always possible. Large, peaked V waves should alert one to the possibility of acute mitral regurgitation (see Chapter 20). In the coronary care unit (CCU) the mean PCWP (integrated electrically by the equipment) is conventionally recorded. One should remember that there are other causes of elevated PCWP besides left ventricular dysfunction (e.g., mitral stenosis). Patients with chronic lung disease should have normal PCWP unless there is associated left ventricular disease. However, patients with chronic obstructive pulmonary disease tend to have marked respiratory variation in their

PCWP tracings. The highest level during expiration and the lowest level during inspiration should be obtained and these values averaged.

The following are the indications for insertion of arterial lines, PA catheters, or both. Clearly, each patient should be considered individually before the decision for invasive monitoring is made.

1. Cardiogenic shock or hypotension (see Chapter 21).
2. Severe left ventricular failure with pulmonary edema, mitral regurgitation, and/or ventricular septal rupture (see Chapters 19 and 20).
3. Significant and persistent sinus tachycardia (120 to 150 beat per minute). Such patients may have low filling pressures; the heart rate may be lowered in such patients by adequate volume expansion (see Chapters 17 and 19).
4. Suspected right ventricular infarction (see Chapter 26).

NB: Although the flow-directed balloon-tipped catheter is used extensively in intensive care units, catheterization laboratories, operating rooms, and emergency wards, major complications (including fatal ones) have been reported with its use. If the correlation between PCWP and pulmonary end-diastolic pressure is good in any one patient, the latter should be used to monitor left ventricular filling pressure to keep "wedge" time to a minimum. This seems to be particularly important if the PA pressure is high. A number of retrospective studies have suggested increased mortality rates in patients who receive a bedside pulmonary arterial catheter. Considerable debate continues concerning the advisability of bedside hemodynamic monitoring in patients with AMI. Given this discussion, it seems reasonable to restrict hemodynamic monitoring to the most critically ill MI patients.

PROTOCOL: PULMONARY ARTERIAL CATHETERIZATION

1. Insertion of the flow-directed catheter can be accomplished percutaneously through the right femoral vein using the same modified Seldinger technique as described for pacemakers (see Chapter 18). Many institutions prefer to insert these catheters by antecubital vein cutdown or percutaneous subclavian or internal jugular vein routes. There is an increased risk of deep venous thrombosis when the femoral vein route is employed.

2. The procedure should be discussed with the patient or next of kin and informed consent obtained. A note should be placed in the patient's chart explaining the indications.

3. It is important that the pressure equipment be calibrated, flushed, and "ready to go" before the catheter is introduced into the PA.

4. The larger 7F catheter is preferred because of the ease of withdrawing blood samples for oxygen saturation determination.

5. Although fluoroscopy is not necessary when this catheter is introduced into the PA and PCW positions, the equipment should be ready on standby in case of need. Appropriate catheter position is easily checked with fluoroscopy.

6. It is important to test the integrity of the balloon (before introducing it into the vein) by inflating it under water with 0.8 ml of air.

7. Once the catheter is introduced into the vein, it should be advanced to the right atrium, which is usually a distance of about 35 cm if the arm or leg is used (markers are placed at 10-cm distances along the shaft of the catheter). When the catheter tip is in the thorax, the patient's cough will produce marked deflections in the pressure tracing.

8. Once the tip of the catheter is in the thorax, 0.8 to 1.5 ml of air (in the 7F catheter) is introduced into the balloon.

9. The catheter is then gently advanced through the right atrium, right ventricle, and PA to the PCW position, each chamber position being documented by the characteristic pressure tracing. Fluoroscopic guidance can also be employed.

10. After passage of the catheter into the PCW position, the balloon should be deflated. The time period during which the wedge pressure is recorded must be kept to a minimum so as to lessen the stress on the PA wall and to prevent pulmonary infarction, PA rupture, or both. This is especially important in patients with chronic pulmonary arterial hypertension. The catheter, when not measuring PCW pressure, should rest in the PA, verified by a PA pressure tracing.

11. When inflating the balloon to record PCW pressure, one should slowly add air to the balloon until the pressure tracing changes from the PA to the PCW configu-

ration. If considerably less air is needed to obtain a PCW pressure than that recommended on the shaft of the catheter, one can assume that the catheter has migrated too far into the wedge position, and it should be gradually pulled back into a position where full or nearly full balloon inflation volume is needed to record wedge pressure. It should be kept in mind that inflation must be performed slowly and stopped when the change from PA to PCW pressure is noted. Should the catheter tip migrate to the PCW position for prolonged periods of time, pulmonary infarction may be induced. Frequent monitoring of the catheter tip is therefore necessary. If fluoroscopy is not used, a chest radiograph should be obtained following the procedure to check the catheter position. The PCW and PA end-diastolic pressures are usually within a few millimeters of mercury of each other.

12. Fluid should not be used to inflate the balloon, since it may be irretrievable. To prevent unintentional injection of fluids, it is recommended that the inflation syringe be kept constantly attached to the balloon lumen.

13. A constant infusion through the catheter lumen should be maintained at all times, and small amounts of heparin (10,000 U/1000 ml of infusate) should be added to this solution.

14. The balloon should be deflated when the catheter is removed.

15. The cardiac index by the Fick principle is determined as follows:
    a. Simultaneous or nearly simultaneous pulmonary arterial and systemic arterial blood samples are obtained in heparinized syringes for blood gas analysis.
    b. The oxygen content of these samples is calculated as described in the Protocol in Chapter 20.
    c. The patient's total body oxygen consumption is determined with a Douglas bag and the help of the catheterization laboratory, or it is obtained from the table in Appendix IV.
    d. The cardiac index is calculated from the following formula: Cardiac index (L/min/m^2) = oxygen consumption index systemic ÷ systemic arterial O_2 content – pulmonary arterial O_2 content. The normal cardiac index is generally 2.8 L/min/m^2 or

more. Normal pulmonary arterial oxygen saturation is 75%, and normal systemic arterial oxygen
saturation is 95%. The technique for systemic arterial pressure monitoring varies. In most CCUs the
radial, brachial, or femoral arteries are used. The
last two routes are preferred because the catheter
tip is closest to the central aorta. Systemic arterial
lines allow one to obtain frequent recordings of systemic blood pressure and blood samples for arterial
blood gas analysis.

A mean systemic arterial pressure of 70 mm Hg is
required to maintain adequate glomerular filtration. A peak
systolic pressure of 90 mm Hg may be appropriate for a
given patient provided that there are no clinical signs of
hypoperfusion. The blood pressure determined by cuff may
underestimate the actual intra-arterial pressure by 10 mm
Hg or more.

PROTOCOL: ARTERIAL CATHETERIZATION

1. Percutaneous insertion of small Teflon catheters into
   the radial, brachial, or femoral arteries can usually be
   accomplished by means of the Seldinger technique. This
   technique has been previously described for venous
   catheterization (see Chapter 18). Several differences
   should be noted between the venous and arterial
   Seldinger techniques:
   a. In the arterial Seldinger technique, the Seldinger
      needle is aimed directly at the arterial pulsation.
   b. No syringe is placed on the Seldinger needle during
      withdrawal. A large (1- to 2-in. arc), pulsating
      stream of blood emerges from the end of the needle
      when its tip is completely within the lumen of the
      artery.
   c. No attempt should be made to thread the guide
      wire through the Seldinger needle unless a pul-
      sating stream of blood is emerging from the end of
      the needle.
2. Once the Teflon catheter is inserted over the guide wire
   and into the artery, it should be well secured to prevent
   accidental dislodgment.
3. Peripheral pulses (beyond a brachial or femoral arterial
   catheterization) should be monitored daily and the
   catheter withdrawn if signs of arterial insufficiency
   develop.

4. The arterial line should be continuously flushed by means of a one-way valve and a pressurized plastic bag containing a heparinized (10,000 U/1000 ml 5% D/W) infusate.

BIBLIOGRAPHY

Connors, A.F., Jr., Speroff, T., Dawson, N.V., et al. The effectiveness of right heart catheterization in the initial care of critically ill patients. *J.A.M.A.* 276:889–897, 1996.

Gardner, R.M., Schwartz, R., Wong, H.C., and Burk, J.P. Percutaneous indwelling radial-artery catheters for monitoring cardiovascular function—Prospective study of the risk of thrombus and infection. *N. Engl. J. Med.* 290: 1227–1231, 1974.

Gore, J.M., Alpert, J.S., Benotti, J.R., Kotilainen, P.W., and Haffajee, C.I. *Handbook of Hemodynamic Monitoring.* Boston: Little, Brown, 1985.

Kearney, T.J., and Shabot, M.M. Pulmonary artery rupture associated with the Swan-Ganz catheter. *Chest* 108: 1349–1352, 1995.

Mueller, H.S., Chatterjee, K., Davis, K.B., et al. Present use of bedside right heart catheterization in patients with cardiac disease. *J. Am. Coll. Cardiol.* 32:840–864, 1998.

Pape, L.A., Haffajee, C.I., Markis, J.E., et al. Fatal pulmonary hemorrhage after use of the flow-directed balloon-tipped catheter. *Ann. Intern. Med.* 90:344–347, 1979.

Swan, H.J.C., Ganz, W., Forrester, J., Marcus, H., Diamond, G., and Chonette, D. Catheterization of the heart in man with the use of a flow-directed balloon-tipped catheter. *N. Engl. J. Med.* 283:447–451, 1970.

30

Cardiac Catheterization, Percutaneous Coronary Arterial Angioplasty, and Cardiac Surgery

Urgent or emergency cardiac catheterization, angioplasty, and/or cardiac surgery are commonly employed in patients with acute myocardial infarction (AMI). These procedures are associated with higher risk in patients with acute infarction as compared with patients with remote infarcts (at least 4 to 6 weeks after infarction). However, in many critically ill patients, angioplasty or cardiac surgery can be lifesaving. Counterpulsation devices (see Chapter 28) enable the physician to stabilize many of these critically ill patients and thus gain time for the consideration of cardiac catheterization and surgery.

Patients in the following diagnostic categories may be candidates for urgent or emergent catheterization, angioplasty, and/or surgery. Counterpulsation may be employed before, during, and after catheterization in such patients. In addition, counterpulsation may be required for several days (occasionally longer) following cardiac surgery.

1. Cardiogenic shock (see Chapter 21). Some patients (40% to 50%) with cardiogenic shock can be salvaged by means of coronary angioplasty or coronary artery bypass. Unless a mechanical defect such as mitral regurgitation or ventricular septal rupture can be corrected during surgery, mortality is high (40% to 60%). Angioplasty should be performed as early as possible in the shock state, preferably within 12 to 18 hours of the onset of shock (see Chapter 30).

2. Unstable angina pectoris refractory to medical management following infarction (see Chapter 24) or in the absence of infarction (see Chapter 23). These two groups include patients who have angina with minimal or no exertion despite hospitalization on optimal medical regimens. Angioplasty or coronary bypass surgery is often indicated. Mortality is inversely proportional to the adequacy of left ventricular function: the more normal the left ventricular function, the lower the mortality. Angioplasty or bypass surgery is usually successful in stabi-

lizing such patients by improving myocardial blood flow. Many of the patients in this category will be on large doses of beta blockers, nitrates, and/or calcium channel blockers. Therapy should be continued right up to the beginning of the surgical procedure. Should it be necessary to discontinue therapy for any reason, an increase in anginal frequency or intensity should prompt initiation of intravenous nitroglycerin therapy.

3. Severe left ventricular failure with acute mitral regurgitation or ventricular septal rupture (see Chapters 19 and 20). Appropriate surgical procedures in selected patients include various combinations of coronary bypass grafting, mitral valve replacement, and ventricular septal repair. Surgery should be performed as soon as possible after the development of one of these complications or 4 to 6 weeks later.

4. Recurrent, life-threatening ventricular arrhythmias (e.g., ventricular tachycardia or fibrillation) refractory to medical therapy. Selected patients with this devastating problem have responded to coronary artery bypass grafting, at times in combination with aneurysmectomy. Careful electrophysiologic study of the patient in the electrophysiology laboratory and at the time of open-heart surgery increases the likelihood of successful surgical extirpation of malignant ventricular arrhythmias. Most of these patients are treated with automatic implantable cardioverter/defibrillator (AICD) devices.

5. Some physicians advocate emergency coronary artery bypass grafting for patients with AMI. These clinicians argue for early reestablishment of myocardial blood flow as soon as possible after coronary thrombosis. Patients are catheterized as soon as they are identified in the emergency department. They undergo coronary bypass grafting shortly thereafter, often within 4 to 8 hours after the onset of AMI. This aggressive surgical approach to patients with AMI is effective in selected patients in centers dedicated to this type of therapy. Urgent thrombolysis (pharmacological or by angioplasty) is more commonly performed. Such therapy is discussed in Chapter 13.

BIBLIOGRAPHY
Allen, B.S., Rosenkranz, E., Buckburg, G.D., et al. Studies on prolonged acute regional ischemia: VI. Myocardial infarction with left ventricular power failure: A medical/

surgical emergency requiring urgent revascularization with maximal protection of remote muscle. *J. Thorac. Cardiovasc. Surg.* 98:691–703, 1989.

Bates, E.R., et al. Comparative long-term effects of coronary artery bypass surgery and percutaneous transluminal coronary angioplasty on regional coronary flow reserve. *Circulation* 72:833–839, 1985.

Berg, R., Jr., Selinger, L.L., Leonard, J.J., Grunwald, R.P., and O'Grady, W.P. Immediate coronary artery bypass for acute evolving myocardial infarction. *J. Thorac. Cardiovasc. Surg.* 81:493–497, 1981.

Berger, P.B., Holmes, D.R., Stebbins, A.L., et al. Impact of an aggressive invasive catheterization and revascularization strategy on mortality in patients with cardiogenic shock in the GUSTO-I trial. *Circulation* 96:122–127, 1997.

Boden, W.E., O'Rourke, R.A., Crawford, M.H., et al. Outcomes in patients with acute non-Q-wave myocardial infarction randomly assigned to an invasive as compared with a conservative management strategy. *N. Engl. J. Med.* 338:1785–1792, 1998.

DeFeyter, P.J., et al. Emergency coronary angioplasty in refractory unstable angina. *N. Engl. J. Med.* 313:342–346, 1985.

Keen, W.D., Savage, M.P., Fischman, D.L., et al. Comparison of coronary angiographic findings during the first six hours of non-Q-wave and Q-wave myocardial infarction. *Am. J. Cardiol.* 74:324–328, 1994.

Phillips, S.J., Zeff, R.H., Skinner, J.R., Toon, K.S., Grignon, A., and Kongtahworn, C. Reperfusion protocol and results in 738 patients with evolving myocardial infarction. *Ann. Thorac. Surg.* 41:119–125, 1986.

Rothbaum, D.A., Linnemeier, T.J., Landin, R.J., et al. Emergency percutaneous transluminal coronary angioplasty in acute myocardial infarction: A 3 year experience. *J. Am. Coll. Cardiol.* 10:264–272, 1987.

Stone, G.W. Direct coronary angioplasty in acute myocardial infarction: Outcome in patients with single vessel disease. *J. Am. Coll. Cardiol.* 15:534–543, 1990.

31

Cardiac Rehabilitation and Follow-Up of Patients after Discharge from the Hospital

In-hospital rehabilitation seldom occurs today because of ever-shortening hospitalizations for acute myocardial infarction (AMI). Many patients are hospitalized for only 4 to 6 days and then directed to a phase II outpatient program. Only 15% of eligible patients in the United States receive cardiac rehabilitation services. Nevertheless, prior to discharge, patients should be educated about risk-factor reduction, especially smoking cessation, exercise prescription, cholesterol management, blood pressure control, diabetes mellitus management, weight control, and medication compliance. Questions regarding sexual activity should be addressed. Most patients are now discharged home with prescriptions for aspirin, beta-adrenergic blockers, statins, sublingual nitroglycerin, and angiotensin-converting enzyme inhibitors. A formal risk assessment based on an exercise stress test is useful in identifying low-risk patients and candidates for more invasive testing. Many patients will have undergone cardiac catheterization, including angioplasty and stenting. They will need advice regarding return to work, physical activity limits, medications, and so on.

Psychological factors may become important. Patients go through periods of anxiety, denial, and depression, and these mood disorders, though considered trivial by some physicians, may have an important influence on survival.

Low risk is characterized by:

1. Normal LV function
2. No recurrent ischemia at rest or with exercise
3. No complex arrhythmias at rest or with exertion
4. Uncomplicated AMI
5. Functional capacity ≥ 6 metabolic units during exercise 3 or more weeks after AMI. To characterize risk, a low-level exercise test or stress test without exercise should be performed (e.g. dobutamine echocardiogram or dipyridamole thallium) at about 2 to 4 weeks after the AMI.

PROTOCOL
1. Patient education begins during or shortly after the patient leaves the coronary care unit (CCU). The pri-

mary emphasis is on risk-factor control, exercise prescription, and knowledge of medications.

2. Ambulation can be started as soon as the patient leaves the CCU, but isometric exercises should be avoided. Sexual activity should not resume until a stress test is completed.

3. Patients should undergo a sub-maximal symptom limited exercise test at 2 to 4 weeks after the AMI if clinically stable. Patients who are unable to exercise should have a dobutamine echocardiogram or dipyridamole thallium test done to exclude provocable ischemia. If ischemia occurs and is more than minimal or if ventricular arrhythmias are induced, coronary angiography should be considered.

BIBLIOGRAPHY

Alpert, J.S. *The Heart Attack Handbook: A Guide to Treatment, Recovery, and Staying Well.* Boston: Little, Brown, 2nd ed., 1984.

Davidson, D.M., and DeBusk, R.F. Prognostic value of a single exercise test 3 weeks after uncomplicated myocardial infarction. *Circulation* 61:236–242, 1980.

DeBusk, R.F., Convertino, V.A., Hung, J. and Goldwater, D. Exercise conditioning in middle-aged men after 10 days of bed rest. *Circulation* 68:245–250, 1983.

DeBusk, R.F., Houston, N., Haskell, W., Fry, G., and Parker, M. Exercise training soon after myocardial infarction. *Am. J. Cardiol.* 44:1223–1229, 1979.

Erb, B.D., Fletcher, G.F., and Sheffield, L.T. Standards for supervised cardiovascular exercise maintenance programs. Report of the subcommittee on exercise/rehabilitation target activity group. *Circulation* 62:669A–672A, 1980.

Fox, S.M., Naughton, J.P., and Gorman, P.A. Physical activity and cardiovascular health. The exercise prescription: Intensity and duration. *Mod. Concepts Cardiovasc. Dis.* 41:21–24, 1972.

Fox, S.M., Naughton, J.P., and Gorman, P.A. Physical activity and cardiovascular health. The exercise prescription: Frequency and type of activity. *Mod. Concepts Cardiovasc. Dis.* 41:25–30, 1972.

Fuller, C.M., Raizner, A.E., Verani, M.S., Nahorek, P.A., Chahine, R.A., McEntee, C.W., and Miller, R.R. Early postmyocardial infarction treadmill stress testing. An accurate predictor of multivessel coronary disease and subsequent cardiac events. *Ann. Intern. Med.* 94:734–739, 1981.

Furberg, C.D., Friedewald, W.T., and Eberlein, K.A., eds. Proceedings of the workshop on implications of recent beta blocker trails for post-myocardial infarction patients. *Circulation* (Suppl. I)96:I-1–I-111, 1983.

Kallio, V., Hamalainen, H., Hakkila, J., et al. Reduction in sudden deaths by a multifactorial intervention programme after acute myocardial infarction. *Lancet* 2:1091–1094, 1979.

Scheuer, J., Greenberg, M.A., and Zohman, L.R. Exercise training in patients with coronary artery disease. *Mos. Concepts Cardiovasc. Dis.* 47:85–90, 1978.

Schwartz, K.M., Turner, J.D., Sheffield, L.T., Roitman, D.I., Kansal, S., Papapietro, S.E., Mantle, J.A., Rackley, C.E., Russell, R.O., Jr., and Rogers, W.J. Limited exercise testing soon after myocardial infarction. Correlation with early coronary and left ventricular angiography. *Ann. Intern. Med.* 94:727–734, 1981.

Starling, M.R., Crawford, M.H., Kennedy, G.T., and O'Rourke, R.A. Exercise testing early after myocardial infarction: Predictive value for subsequent unstable angina and death. *Am. J. Cardiol.* 46:909–914, 1980.

Verani, M.S., Hartung, G.H., Hoepfel-Harris, J., Welton, D.E., Pratt, C.M., Miller, R.R., and DelVentura, L.A. Effects of exercise training on the left ventricular performance and myocardial perfusion in patients with coronary artery disease. *Am. J. Cardiol.* 47:797–803, 1981

Wenger, N.K. *Exercise and the Heart.* Philadelphia: Davis, 1978.

32

Hyperlipidemia in the Patient with Myocardial Infarction

Compelling scientific evidence now demonstrates that reduction of risk factors in patients with coronary artery disease (CAD) and peripheral vascular disease improves long-term survival and quality of life, decreases the need for interventional procedures such as coronary bypass surgery and angioplasty, and reduces the incidence of subsequent myocardial infarction (MI). Particularly important is control of hyperlipidemia, especially hypercholesterolemia.

Much of the data supporting these recommendations has been obtained from post-MI patients, but the results can be generalized to all patients with atherosclerotic disease regardless of the vascular territory affected. Modest regression (10% to 15%) of atherosclerotic vascular disease can be achieved with meticulous reduction in serum cholesterol. Close control of serum glucose in patients with diabetes mellitus can also help to regulate serum lipid levels, with consequent reduction in clinical vascular events in post-MI individuals. Antihyperlipidemic therapy seeks to lower low-density lipoprotein (LDL) cholesterol and/or triglycerides while not affecting or raising high-density lipoprotein (HDL) cholesterol. LDL cholesterol plays a major role in the development of atherosclerosis in both men and women, although women develop clinical atherosclerotic disease an average of 10 to 15 years later than men.

1. Diagnosis. Serum cholesterol levels should be measured in all MI patients on admission. These values approximate the patient's usual lipid results. Measurements should quantitate both LDL and HDL cholesterol as well as total cholesterol and triglyceride levels.

   In post-MI patients high-, borderline-, and low-risk values are lower than those designated for individuals without known vascular disease. Thus, LDL cholesterol higher than 130 mg/dl is considered high risk, values of 100 to 130 mg/dl are borderline high risk, and values below 100 mg/dl are desirable. Triglyceride values are also determined and used to guide therapy: triglyceride levels below 160 mg/dl are desirable.

2. Therapy. Diet and various drugs are used to treat hyperlipidemia. It is particularly important that diabetic

hyperlipidemic patients receive aggressive lipid-lowering therapy since they are at particularly high risk for recurrent MI.

a. Diets used to treat hyperlipidemia. Two levels of diet are used to treat hyperlipidemia, Step I and Step II. The Step I diet is less rigorous than the Step II diet. The Step I diet contains 30% or fewer of its calories as fat, with 8% to 10% of total calories as saturated fat. Cholesterol intake is reduced to less than 300 mg daily. In the Step II diet, saturated fat is reduced to less than 7% of calories and cholesterol intake is reduced below 200 mg daily. Detailed dietary information is available from nutritionists or in the Second Report of the Expert Panel on Detection, Evaluation, and Treatment of High Blood Cholesterol in Adults (see the bibliography at the end of this chapter).

b. Drugs used to treat hyperlipidemia.

   (1) Bile-acid sequestrants. The major effect of bile-acid sequestrants is to lower LDL cholesterol. The sequestrants are anion-exchange resins that bind bile acids in the intestinal lumen. They thereby interrupt the enterohepatic circulation of bile acids and promote conversion of cholesterol to bile acids in the liver. Reducing liver cholesterol content stimulates the formation of LDL receptors, which reduces serum cholesterol levels. The two commonly employed bile acid sequestrants are cholestyramine and colestipol. Their use is associated with significant gastrointestinal side effects (e.g., constipation, bloating, nausea, and flatulence). The usual dose of cholestyramine is 4 to 16 g/day; the usual dose of colestipol is 5 to 20 g/day.

   (2) Nicotinic acid. This agent lowers all serum lipid and lipoprotein values when given in large doses. Nicotinic acid reduces the production of very low density lipoproteins (VLDLs) in the liver, which in turn lowers serum triglyceride and LDL cholesterol levels. Nicotinic acid also raises serum HDL cholesterol levels. Nicotinic acid comes in two forms, crystalline (short-acting) and sustained-release capsules. The usual dose is 1.5 to 3 g/day for crystalline nicotinic acid and 1 to 2 g/day for the sustained-release

formulation. Adverse reactions are common and include flushing, hyperglycemia, hyperuricemia, gastrointestinal complaints, and hepatic toxicity. Serum hepatic function tests should be monitored during therapy. Flushing is at times countered by administering one to two aspirin tablets per day.

(3) HMG-CoA reductase inhibitors ("statins"). These agents are the most effective drugs currently available for lowering serum cholesterol. They inhibit the enzyme HMG-CoA reductase, a key, rate-limiting component in the biochemical pathway for the synthesis of cholesterol. Inhibition of this pathway results in increased synthesis of LDL receptors, which lowers serum cholesterol. Commonly employed HMG-CoA reductase inhibitors include: lovastatin, pravastatin, simvastatin, fluvastatin, and cerivastatin. Side effects include dyspepsia, flatus, constipation, and abdominal pain and cramps as well as hepatic toxicity. Serum hepatic function tests should be monitored during therapy. The usual doses are lovastatin, 10 to 80 mg/day; pravastatin, 10 to 40 mg/day; simvastatin, 5 to 40 mg/day; fluvastatin, 10 to 40 mg/day.

(4) Fibric acid derivatives. There are currently three fibric acid derivatives available in the United States, gemfibrozil, fenofibrate, and clofibrate (Atromid). Gemfibrozil (Lopid) is the most commonly used product. These agents increase the activity of the enzyme lipoprotein lipase, which enhances catabolism of VLDLs and intermediate density lipoproteins (IDLs) and reduce serum triglyceride levels. HDL cholesterol levels are increased by fibric acid derivative therapy. Side effects include gastrointestinal complaints and increased gallstone formation. The usual dose of gemfibrozil is 600 mg b.i.d.; the usual dose of clofibrate is 50 mg t.i.d. or q.i.d.

PROTOCOL

1. The patient's lipid profile on admission to the hospital is usually an accurate reflection of his or her daily lipid value. Serum cholesterol decreases rapidly over the first 1 to 3 days following hospitalization. Consequently, lipid

values determined after admission are of less value to the clinician.

2. All post-MI patients should adhere to a Step II diet. In addition, it is our practice to initiate lipid-lowering therapy on the second or third hospital day even in patients with "normal" cholesterol—e.g., total cholesterol = 190 mg/dl and LDL cholesterol = 110 mg/dl. These allegedly normal values are almost certainly too high and have led to the development of coronary arterial atherosclerosis.

3. If cholesterol levels are elevated and serum triglyceride levels are less than 200 mg/dl, patients should be treated with a statin, a bile acid sequestrant, or niacin. A statin is usually the preferred therapy.

4. If cholesterol levels are elevated and serum triglyceride levels are between 200 and 400 mg/dl, patients should be treated with either a statin or niacin.

5. If cholesterol levels are elevated and serum triglyceride levels are greater than 400 mg/dl, patients should be treated with combination therapy (niacin, fibric acid derivative, statin).

6. In all patients, if monotherapy fails to lower LDL cholesterol to the desirable range, combination therapy should be considered.

7. In all post-MI patients, the physician seeks to lower LDL cholesterol levels below 100 mg/dl.

8. Fasting lipid levels should be rechecked 4 weeks after initiating therapy.

9. Regular aerobic exercise is advised for all hyperlipidemic patients. A minimum of 30 to 60 minutes of exercise 3 to 4 times per week is encouraged. Maximum benefit probably occurs at 5 to 6 hours per week.

BIBLIOGRAPHY

Blakenhorn, D.H., Nessium, S.A., Johnson, R.L., Sanmarco, M.E., Azen, S.P., and Cashin-Hemphill, L. Beneficial effects of colestipol niacin therapy on coronary atherosclerosis and coronary venous bypass grafts. *J.A.M.A.* 257: 3233–3240, 1987.

Cashin-Hemphill, L., Mack, W.J., Pogoda, M.J., Sanmarco, M.E., Azen, S.P., and Blankenhorn, D.H. Beneficial effects of colestipol-niacin on coronary atherosclerosis. *J.A.M.A.* 264:3013–3017, 1990.

Furberg, C.D., Adams, H.P. Jr., Applegate, W.B., et al. Effect of lovastatin on early carotid atherosclerosis and cardiovascular events. *Circulation* 90:1679, 1994.

Gould, A.L., Rossouw, J.E., Santanello, N.C., et al. Cholesterol reduction yields clinical benefit—A new look at old data. *Circulation* 91:2274, 1995.

Kjekshus, J., Pedersen, T.R., and Pyoraia K. for the 4S Group. Impact of hypertension, diabetes and smoking on the effect of simvastatin on coronary events in coronary heart disease patients. *Circulation* 92(suppl 1):86–94, 1995.

Kwiterovich, P.O. Jr. State-of-the-art update and review: Clinical trials of lipid-lowering agents. *Am. J. Cardiol.* 82: 3U–17U, 1998.

National Cholesterol Education Program. Second Report of the Expert Panel on Detection, Evaluation, and Treatment of High Blood Cholesterol in Adults (adult treatment panel II). *Circulation* 89:1329, 1994.

Ornish, D., Brown, S.E., Scherwitz, L.W., et al. Can lifestyle changes reverse coronary heart disease? *Lancet* 336: 129–133, 1990.

Prevention of cardiovascular events and death with pravastatin in patients with coronary heart disease and a broad range of initial cholesterol levels. The Long-Term Intervention with Pravastatin in Ischaemic Disease (LIPID) Study Group. *N. Engl. J. Med.* 339:1349–1357, 1998.

Sacks, F.M., Pfeffer, M.A., Moye, L.A., et al. for the Cholesterol and Recurrent Events Trial Investigators. The effect of pravastatin on coronary events after myocardial infarction in patients with average cholesterol level. *N. Engl. J. Med.* 335:1001–1009, 1996.

Scandinavian Simvastatin Survival Study Group. Randomized trial of cholesterol lowering in 4444 patients with coronary heart disease: the Scandinavian Simvastatin Survival Study (4S). *Lancet* 344:1383–1389, 1994.

Schler, G., Hambrecht, R., Schlierf, G., et al. Regular physical exercise and low-fat diet: Effects on progression of coronary artery disease. *Circulation* 86:1–11, 1992.

Superko, H.R., and Krauss, R.M. Coronary artery disease regression—Convincing evidence for the benefit of aggressive lipoprotein management. *Circulation* 90:1056, 1994.

Waters, D., Higginson, L., Gladstone, P. et al. Effect of monotherapy with HMG-CoA reductase inhibitor on the progression of coronary atherosclerosis is assessed by serial quantitative arteriography: The Canadian Coronary Atherosclerosis Intervention Trial. *Circulation* 89:959–968, 1994.

Watts, G.F., Lewis, B., Brunt, J.N., et al. Effects on coronary artery disease of lipid-lowering diet, or diet plus cholestyramine, in the St. Thomas' Atherosclerosis Repression Study (STARS). *Lancet* 339:563–569, 1992.

33

Sexual Activity after Myocardial Infarction

Sexual dysfunction is common in patients after myocardial infarction (MI). As many as three out of four men report either impotence or a marked decrease in libido following MI. Although fewer data are available on women, it appears that they also exhibit a similar decrease in sexual activity after MI. Such sexual dysfunction can be organic in origin, caused by medication, anginal episodes, or low cardiac output or blood pressure. However, in the majority of postinfarction patients, sexual dysfunction is the end result of a combination of organic and psychological factors such as anxiety, depression, and poor self-image. These psychological responses are very common in post-MI patients and frequently result in considerable anguish. It is therefore not surprising that sexual difficulties often develop.

Physicians may be reluctant to discuss sexual functioning with their patients. Reasons include embarrassment, lack of knowledge concerning the effects of sexual activity on cardiac physiology, and inexperience in sexual counseling.

1. Cardiovascular physiology of sexual intercourse. During coitus, normal men and women of all ages experience an increase in blood pressure of as much as 30 to 80 mm Hg systolic and 20 to 50 mm Hg diastolic as well as a peak heart rate of up to 140 to 180 beats per minute. Older persons probably experience heart rate and blood pressure increases that are at the lower end of these ranges. Even these lower increases can significantly elevate the product of heart rate and blood pressure—an indirect index of myocardial oxygen consumption or metabolism. Such a marked increase in myocardial metabolic demand may be hazardous in a patient with severe ischemic heart disease. Fortunately, the increases in heart rate and blood pressure in post-MI patients who engage in *conjugal* sexual intercourse are considerably smaller than those observed in normal, younger individuals. During marital intercourse, post-MI patients usually achieve peak heart rates of 120 to 130 beats per minute and peak blood pressures of about 160/90 mm Hg. Since heart rate and blood pressure increases dur-

ing intercourse appear to be smaller in middle-aged patients than in normal younger men and women and since these hemodynamic determinants of myocardial oxygen consumption are also smaller during conjugal than during nonconjugal relations, it is reasonable to expect that the myocardial metabolic demand during conjugal sex will be considerably less in post-MI patients than in normal young persons.

2. Clinical observations. The rather modest increases in myocardial oxygen consumption that occur in post-MI patients during marital sexual relations are similar to the demands placed on the heart by routine daily activities such as climbing stairs or walking briskly. Many patients can tolerate such activities soon after MI.

   Patients and their spouses often harbor unfounded fears that sexual activity will precipitate another MI or even sudden death. Such events, appropriately termed *morte d'amour,* appear to be unusual. In one report from Japan, only 0.6% of studied sudden deaths occurred during coitus. It is of interest, moreover, that in this series of cases 80% of the deaths that did occur during or immediately after intercourse were associated with extramarital sex. Although some patients with ischemic heart disease develop angina or arrhythmias during intercourse, it appears that such symptoms are unusual and of minor clinical significance.

3. Effects of therapy. Because beta-blocking agents such as propranolol and vasodilators such as isosorbide dinitrate decrease myocardial oxygen demand during exercise and coitus, they may ameliorate or abolish angina or arrhythmias induced by sexual activity in post-MI patients. Those individuals who continue to experience angina during coitus despite therapy with anti-anginal agents can still experience angina-free intercourse by taking a sublingual nitroglycerin a minute or two before initiating sexual activity. Physical conditioning such as that resulting from a well-designed cardiac rehabilitation program also results in a decrease in myocardial oxygen demand during coitus. In men, however, beta-blocking agents and antihypertensive drugs may cause impotence. This drug-induced impotence is often a matter of great concern to the patient and requires careful counseling and even alteration of the medical regimen to allow for the use of sildenafil (Viagra).

4. Sexual counseling guidelines. The following guidelines should be useful in helping patients to reestablish normal sexual relations after myocardial infarction:

    a. It is best to avoid coitus immediately after eating, immediately after drinking alcohol, in an uncomfortably hot or cold environment, just before or after strenuous exercise, when feeling angry or fatigued, and/or when anginal episodes have been occurring at rest or with minimal exertion.

    b. Ample time should be allowed to initiate and consummate coitus.

    c. In resuming sexual activity for the first time after MI, patients should consider the advisability of engaging in intimacy without coitus for the first day or two, adopting gentle, nonathletic coital positions and taking prophylactic sublingual nitroglycerin just before initiating sexual relations unless Viagra is employed.

    Overexertion during coitus may result in excessive sinus tachycardia or other arrhythmias, marked dyspnea, or angina. If such symptoms occur during or immediately after coitus, the physician should consider the possible value of exercise or specific pharmacologic or surgical therapy for ischemic heart disease.

    d. Sildenafil (Viagra) is a selective inhibitor of cyclic GMP phosphodiesterase (type 5), producing smooth muscle relaxation, vasodilatation, and enhanced penile erection. The cardiovascular effects of Viagra are modest in normal individuals, consisting of small decreases in systolic (8 to 10 mm Hg) and diastolic (5 to 6 mm Hg) blood pressure and no change in heart rate. These effects last for approximately 4 hours after ingestion of Viagra. They can be magnified in patients taking any form of nitrate preparation. Indeed, marked hypotension and even death can occur. It is recommended that 24 hours elapse between dosing with Viagra and any form of nitrate.

    Since even modest decreases in blood pressure might be hazardous in patients with severe and unstable ischemic heart disease or marked congestive heart failure, Viagra is considered to be contraindicated in them. In addition, a number of drugs (Table 33-1) compete with Viagra for the cytochrome P450 metabolic pathway; hence either their activity

Table 33-1. Drugs metabolized by or inhibiting Cytochrome P450 3A4

Antibiotic/antifungal agents
  Biaxin (clarithromycin)
  Clotrimazole
  Erythromycin
  Diflucan
  Sporanox
  Ketoconazole
  Miconazole
  Noroxin
  Troleandomycin

Cardiovascular drugs
  Amiodarone
  Norvasc
  Digitoxin
  Diltiazem
  Disopyramide
  Plendil (felodipine)
  DynaCirc (isradipine)
  Cozaar (losartan)
  Nifedipine
  Quinidine
  Verapamil

HMG-CoA reductase inhibitors
  Lipitor (atorvastatin)
  Baycol (cerivastatin)
  Mevacor (lovastatin)
  Zocor (simvastatin)

Central nervous system agents
  Alprazolam
  Carbamazepine
  Prozac (fluoxetine)
  Luvox (fluvoxamine)
  Imipramine
  Serzone (nefazodone)
  Phenobarbital
  Zoloft
  Triazolam

Other drugs
  Acetaminophen
  Hismanal (astemizole)
  Tagamet (cimetidine)
  Propulsid (cisapride)
  Cyclosporine
  Dexamethasone

Table 33-2. Contraindications to Viagra (sildenafil citrate)

Use of Viagra clearly contraindicated:
1. Concurrent use of nitrates
Cardiovascular effects of Viagra may be potentially hazardous for use dependent on individual clinical assessment:
1. Patients with active coronary ischemia who are not taking nitrates (e.g., positive exercise test for ischemia)
2. Patients with congestive heart failure and borderline low blood pressure and borderline low volume status
3. Patients on a complicated multidrug antihypertensive program
4. Patients taking drugs that can prolong the half-life of Viagra

or that of Viagra could be enhanced by concomitant administration of the two agents. Table 33-2 summarizes contraindications to the use of Viagra.

BIBLIOGRAPHY

Cheitlin, M.D., Hutte, A.M. Jr., Brindis, R.G., Ganz, P., Kaul, S., and Russell, R.O. Jr. Use of Sildenafil (Viagra) in patients with cardiovascular disease. *Circulation* 99: 168–177, 1999.

Drory, Y., Fisman, E.Z., Shapira, Y., and Pines, A. Ventricular arrhythmias during sexual activity in patients with coronary artery disease. *Chest* 109:922–924, 1996.

Fox, C.A. Reduction in systolic blood pressure during human coitus by the beta-adrenergic blocking agent, propranolol. *J. Reprod. Fertil.* 22:587–590, 1970.

Haskell, W.L. Restoration and maintenance of physical and psychologic function in patients with ischemic heart disease. *J. Am. Coll. Cardiol.* 12:1117–1121, 1998.

Johnston, B.L., and Fletcher, G.F. Dynamic electrocardiographic recording during sexual activity in recent post-myocardial infarction and revascularization patients. *Am. Heart J.* 98:736–741, 1979.

Nemec, E.D., Mansfield, L., and Kennedy, J.W. Heart rate and blood pressure responses during sexual activity in normal males. *Am. Heart J.* 92:274–277, 1976.

Stein, R.A. The effect of exercise training on heart rate during coitus in the post myocardial infarction patients. *Circulation* 55:738–740, 1977.

Ueno, M. The so-called coition death. *Jpn. J. Legal Med.* 17:333–340, 1963.

Appendix I

Indications, Routes, and Doses of Commonly Employed Medications

Appendix I Table A. Guide for rapid administration of antiarrhythmic drugs (intravenous route)

Drug	Dose	Therapeutic plasma level (µg/ml)	Side effects	Comments
Atropine	0.6–1.0 mg IV as a rapid bolus	—	Sinus tachycardia, glaucomic crisis, urinary retention, psychosis	Occasionally precipitates paradoxical slowing of heart rate or ventricular tachycardia.
Bretylium tosylate	5–10 mg/kg loading dose over 10 min followed by maintenance infusion of 1–2 mg/min	—	Hypotension, nausea, vomiting, transient increase in heart rate and blood pressure	Dose should be reduced in patients with renal failure; patient response may be better when drug is used alone rather than with other antiarrhythmic drugs.
Diltiazem	0.25 mg/kg over 2 min; if inadequate response, repeat after 15 min with 0.35 mg/kg; constant infusion if needed of 5–10 mg/h.	—	Hypotension, heart block, headache	Employed only to slow the ventricular response in atrial fibrillation.
Diphenylhydantoin	50–100 mg IV slowly (50 mg/min) q5min up to 1000 mg. Additional 500 mg on following day.	10–18	Hypotension, 1:1 conduction in atrial flutter, respiratory arrest, idioventricular rhythm, ventricular fibrillation, asystole	Administration IM provides erratic blood levels; toxicity usually seen only after rapid administration.

Appendix I Table A. *Continued*

Drug	Dose	Therapeutic plasma level (µg/ml)	Side effects	Comments
Lidocaine	200-mg IV bolus over 20 min followed by 2–4 mg/min constant infusion. Half the normal loading and maintenance dosage is given for patients with pulmonary edema, shock, and hepatocellular disease.	1.4–6.0	Focal seizures, grand mal seizures, respiratory arrest, dizziness, heart block (usually associated with preexisting abnormal His-Purkinje conduction), sinoatrial arrest	Significant reduction in dose in patients with heart failure, moderate reduction in dose in patients with hepatic disease; no oral form available; no significant myocardial depression; toxicity usually seen at high plasma levels; toxicity at low plasma levels may be caused by metabolites.
Metoprolol	5 mg q5min up to 15 mg	—	Hypotension, bradycardia, prolonged AV conduction and heart block, myocardial depression	Should be used with caution in the presence of heart failure and heart block.
Procainamide	10–12 mg/kg IV slowly (25 mg/min)	4–8	Hypotension, prolonged AV and His-Purkinje conduction	Myocardial toxicity usually occurs only at high plasma levels or after rapid administration.

Drug	Dosage	Therapeutic Level	Side Effects	Comments
Propranolol	1 mg/min IV q3–5 min up to 10 mg	40–85 (ng/ml)	Hypotension, bradycardia, prolonged AV conduction and heart block, myocardial depression, bronchospasm	Should probably not be considered in the presence of severe heart failure; many of the side effects reversed by large doses of isoproterenol.
Verapamil	2.5–10 mg IV bolus; repeated if necessary; may be followed by continuous infusion of 0.005 mg/kg/min	—	Headache, nausea, constipation, hypotension, heart block	Effective only for supraventricular arrhythmias. Do not employ verapamil and beta blockers concomitantly; asystole may result.

Appendix I Table B. Guide for long-term oral administration of antiarrhythmic drugs

Drug	Usual total daily dose*	Frequency of administration	Therapeutic plasma level (μg/ml)	Half-life (h)	Side effects	Comments
Acebutolol	600–1800 mg	q8h	—	3	Same as for propranolol	Selective for β₁ receptors at low dose.
Amiodarone	200–600 mg	Once daily	1–2.5 (steady state)	30–100 days	Tremor, dizziness, pulmonary fibrosis, hyperthyroidism, hypothyroidism, anorexia, nausea, vomiting, alopecia, peripheral neuropathy, insomnia, depression, bradycardia, AV block	Extremely long half-life requires 7–10 days of loading with oral amiodarone; marked enhancement of anticoagulant action of warfarin.
Atenolol	50–100 mg	Once or twice daily	—	—	Same as for propranolol	Selective for β₁ receptors at low dose.
Disopyramide	400–800 mg	q6h	2–5	7	Myocardial depression, hypotension, prolonged AV conduction and heart block, glaucoma, urinary retention, dry mouth, constipation, blurred	Half-life 7 h; reduced dosage in hepatic and renal insufficiency; hypotension can occur in patients with myocarditis or cardiomyopathy, or both;

Metoprolol	100–200 mg	q12h	—	~8	vision, nausea, anorexia	300-mg loading dose advised in patients with life-threatening arrhythmias.
Mexiletine	600–900 mg	tid	0.75–2.0	8–12	Same as for propranolol	Selective for β_1 receptors at low dose.
Nadolol	80–320 mg	Once daily	—	18–24	Same as for tocainide	Similar structure to tocainide.
Phenytoin sodium	300–400 mg	Once daily	10–18	22	Same as for propranolol Nystagmus, ataxia, lethargy, nausea, vertigo, rashes, pseudolymphoma, megaloblastic anemia, peripheral neuropathy, hyperglycemia, seizures	— Half-life higher at higher doses; rate of metabolism affected by many drugs; clinically significant decrease in plasma binding in azotemia and hypoproteinemia, should initiate therapy with 1 g loading dose.

continued

Appendix I Table B. *Continued*

Drug	Usual total daily dose*	Frequency of administration	Therapeutic plasma level (µg/ml)	Half-life (h)	Side effects	Comments
Pindolol	10–30 mg	q12h	—	8–10	Same as for propranolol	Partial beta agonist.
Procainamide	2–6 g	q3–4h	4–8	3–4	Nausea, vomiting, agranulocytosis, lupuslike syndrome, myocardial depression, prolonged AV and His-Purkinje conduction	Toxic myocardial effect usually only at toxic plasma levels; half-life markedly prolonged in renal failure or alkaline urine.
Propranolol	80–320 mg	q6h	40–85 (ng/ml)	3–4.6	Myocardial depression, prolonged AV conduction and heart block, bradycardia, bronchospasm, fatigue, depression, peripheral vascular insufficiency, hyperglycemia, hypoglycemia, alopecia, gastric distention	Active metabolites may play a role in clinical effect; dose chosen empirically; should be tapered slowly in patients with angina; caution needed in patients with cardiac function dependent on sympathetic tone.

Quinidine	1.0–2.4 g	q6h	2.3–5.0 (using double extraction; higher for precipitation assay)	~6	Hypotension, nausea, vomiting, diarrhea, tinnitus, vertigo, prolonged His-Purkinje conduction, rash, fever, thrombocytopenia, hepatic dysfunction, hemolytic anemia, ventricular arrhythmias	Minor gastrointestinal side effects controlled with symptomatic therapy; clinically significant decrease in plasma binding in hypoproteinemia and hepatic disease; myocardial toxicity usually only at toxic plasma levels; accumulation of metabolites in renal disease.
Timolol	10–40 mg	q12h	—	~10	Same as for propranolol	—
Tocainide	600–1800 mg	tid	5–15	14	Light-headedness, tremor, nausea, twitching, diplopia, anorexia, abdominal pain, constipation, rash, fever	Response to tocainide can be predicted by the response of the ventricular arrhythmia to intravenous lidocaine.

* Note: These dosages refer to the cumulative daily doses. Normally, the drugs are administered in divided doses throughout the day.

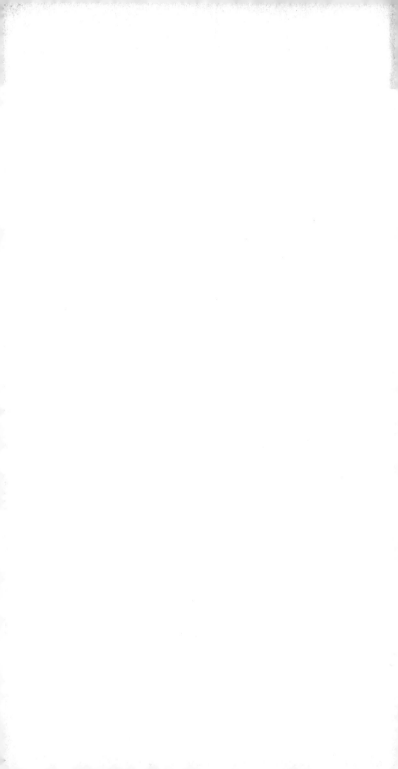

Appendix II

Nomogram for Calculating Body Surface Area from Height and Weight (in m²)

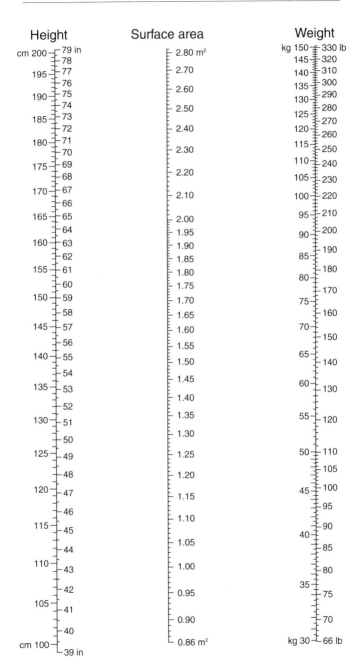

| Height | Surface area | Weight |

Appendix III

Table for Estimating Total Body Oxygen Consumption from Patient's Age, Sex, and Heart Rate

Appendix III   Table A.   Total body oxygen consumption (ml/min) as determined by age, sex, and heart rate

Age	Heart rate (beats/min)						
	<50	51–60	61–70	71–80	81–90	91–100	>100
FEMALES							
<35			128 ± 2.0	136 ± 5.4	136 ± 18.6	136.5 ± 16.4	
36–45		119.7 ± 4.8	124.5 ± 9.5	142.1 ± 9.5	128.4 ± 9.4		
46–55		124.5 ± 8.4	113.1 ± 5.2	117.6 ± 9.2	124.7 ± 6.9	130 ± 12.4	
56–65		104.2 ± 4.5	106 ± 7.9	111.4 ± 5.0	124.5 ± 2.9	134.3 ± 15.1	
66–75		102.1 ± 6.0	105 ± 9.8	124.3 ± 8.8	117.6 ± 10.3	107.7 ± 8.4	
MALES							
<35				158.8 ± 7.3	160 ± 9.4	146 ± 16	
36–45		122.9 ± 4.5	135.3 ± 6.3	138.9 ± 11.4	150.9 ± 8.7	134.4 ± 6.4	133.3 ± 2.5
46–55	119.8 ± 6.8	120.3 ± 2.6	122 ± 3.6	130.6 ± 5.1	134.3 ± 8.6	134.7 ± 5.6	125.5 ± 2.7
56–65	117.9 ± 8.6	121.6 ± 3.5	121 ± 3.8	125 ± 4.4	125.8 ± 7.4	125.4 ± 10.4	125 ± 2.8
66–75	104.8 ± 2.0	113.8 ± 5.7	116.4 ± 6.1	124.1 ± 6.2	124.1 ± 9.2		125.5 ± 19.5

From Crocker RH, Ockene IS, Alpert JS, et al. Determinants of total body oxygen consumption in adults undergoing catheterization. *Cathet Cardiovasc Diagn* 1982;8:363. (Reprinted by permission of Wiley-Liss, a division of John Wiley & Sons, Inc.)

Subject Index

Note: Page numbers followed by f indicate illustrations; those followed by t indicate tables.

A

Abciximab, unstable angina therapy, 135–136, 139
Accelerated idioventricular rhythm
features, 96–97
management, 97, 101
ACE inhibitors. *See* Angiotensin-converting enzyme inhibitors
Acebutolol, dose and side effects, 198t
Acetaminophen, prescription in CCU, 34
ACLS. *See* Advanced Cardiac Life Support
Acute coronary syndrome. *See* Unstable angina
Adenosine, supraventricular tachycardia management, 88, 101
Advanced Cardiac Life Support, equipment and personnel during interhospital transfer, 12–13
Age, prognostic indicator in MI, 15
AIVR. *See* Accelerated idioventricular rhythm
Albumin, blood monitoring following MI, 33
Alprazolam, prescription in CCU, 6, 34
Alteplase, protocol for administration, 64
Amiodarone
atrial fibrillation management, 86–87, 100
dose and side effects, 198t
ventricular tachycardia treatment, 95–96
warfarin interactions, 87
Aneurysm, anterior versus inferior MI, 16t
Angina
dietary heavy metals in precipitation, 21
differential diagnosis, 141

management, 141–142
surgery timing, 142
unstable. *See* Unstable angina
Angioplasty
cardiogenic shock patients, 125, 128
door-to-balloon time, 67
electrocardiogram indications, 45
heart failure patients, 114–115
infarct size effects, 59
rescue
indications for, 18–19, 38, 39, 67
following thrombolysis, 66
stenting, 66–67
thrombolysis with, 66–67
Angiotensin-converting enzyme inhibitors
hypertension treatment following MI, 132
right ventricular infarction management, 156
Anticoagulants
heparin
intravenous, 69
low-molecular-weight heparins, 70–71
indications, 69
platelet glycoprotein antagonists, 69–70
Arrhythmia
accelerated idioventricular rhythm, 96–97, 101
angioplasty or surgical management, 176
atrial fibrillation, 85–87, 100
atrial flutter, 87–88, 100
atrioventricular dissociation, 90, 101
hypothalamic origin of, 5
junctional rhythms, 89–90, 100–101
late hospital phase ventricular arrhythmias, 99
management in patient transport, 11
multifocal atrial tachycardia, 90, 101
paroxysmal atrial tachycardia with block, 89, 100

1st motor